» **Finding your ideal bootcamp, whatever your goals, is just a few steps away. Turn to page 10 to find the perfect plan for you!**

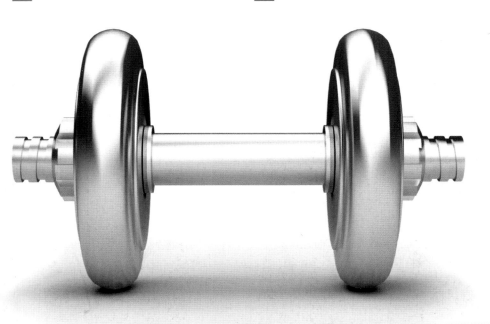

women's
fitness

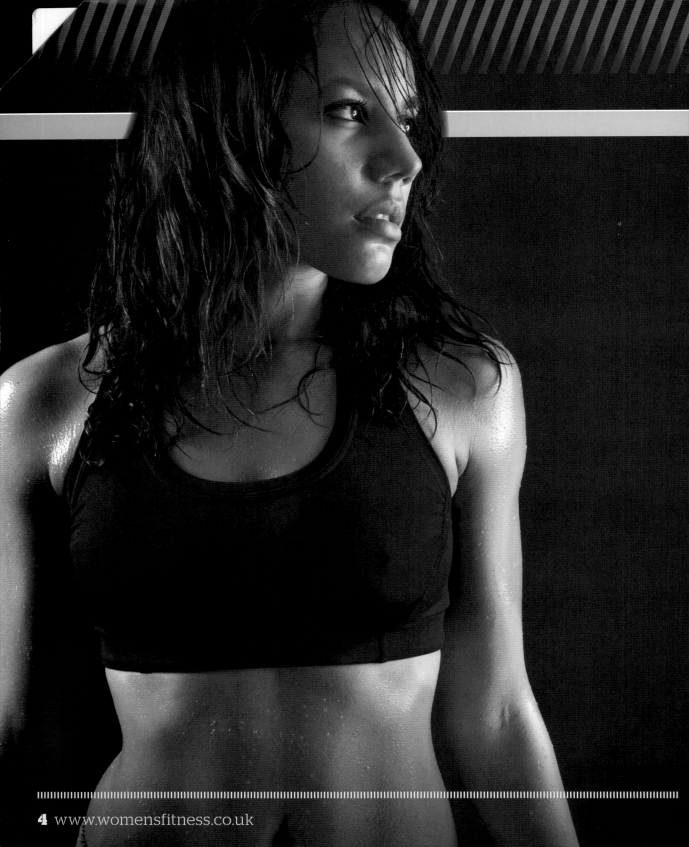

women's fitness

Editor Joanna Knight
Art Director Matt Reynolds
Chief Sub-Editor Penny Carroll
Contributors Amanda Khouv, Louise Pyne, Kristoph Thompson, Lowri Turner
Photography Danny Bird; StockFood; Shutterstock
Model Rachael Tennent, W Athletic, www.wathletic.com

Digital Production Manager Nicky Baker
Management MagBook Dharmesh Mistry
Publisher Dharmesh Mistry
Operations Director Robin Ryan
Advertising Manager Katie Wood
MD of Advertising Julian Lloyd-Evans
Newstrade Director David Barker
Commercial and Retail Director Martin Belson
Chief Operating Officer Brett Reynolds
Group Finance Director Ian Leggett
Chief Executive James Tye
Chairman Felix Dennis

MAG**BOOK**

The MagBook brand is a trademark of Dennis Publishing Ltd. 30 Cleveland St, London W1T 4JD. Company registered in England. All material © Dennis Publishing Ltd, licensed by Felden 2012, and may not be reproduced in whole or part without the consent of the publishers. *Best Body Bootcamp* ISBN 1781060347.

Clothing credits
48-Hour Fat Attack Plan
Adidas top, £20, www.adidas.com; Do shorts, £23, www.dounlimited.com; Adidas Adizero F50 2 trainers, £85, www.adidas.com
1-Week Waist Away Plan
Adidas top, £20, www.adidas.com; Nike leggings, £30, www.nikestore.com; Mizuno Wave Rider trainers, £100, www.sweatshop.co.uk
14-Day Drop A Dress Size Plan
Moving Comfort top, £39.99, www.movingcomfort.co.uk; No Balls leggings, £39, www.noballs.co.uk; New Balance 860V2 trainers, £84.99, www.newbalance.co.uk
4-Week Total Body Blitz Plan
Moving Comfort top, £36.99, www.movingcomfort.co.uk; No Balls shorts, £33, www.noballs.co.uk; K-Swiss Blade Max Stable trainers, £100, www.k-swiss.co.uk
Equipment
Physical Neo-Hex dumbbells and Supaflex X-band, www.physicalcompany.co.uk; Reebok 8kg weight set, www.johnlewis.com; Reebok medicine ball 3kg, Reebok deck, AOK Max Ball and skipping rope, all www.escapefitness.com; Agoy mat, www.agoy.com; Nike mat, www.nikestore.com

Licensing & Syndication
To license this product, please contact Carlotta Serantoni on +44 (0) 20 7907 6550 or email carlotta_serantoni@dennis.co.uk To syndicate content from this product, please contact Anj Dosaj Halai on +44 (0) 20 7907 6132 or email anj_dosaj-halai@dennis.co.uk
Liability
While every care was taken during the production of this MagBook, the publishers cannot be held responsible for the accuracy of the information or any consequence arising from it. Dennis Publishing takes no responsibility for the companies advertising in this MagBook. The paper used within this MagBook is produced from sustainable fibre, manufactured by mills with a valid chain of custody. Printed at BGPrint Ltd.

Always check with your GP before commencing an exercise programme, especially if you have been inactive for a long period of time. Those with a history of high blood pressure or heart disease should obtain medical clearance before undertaking any activity.

Editor's note

>> Bootcamps are one of the best ways to get in shape: they're fast, furious, fun and effective! So whether you want to flatten your tum in a weekend, slim your waist for a special occasion, drop a dress size, or lose up to a stone, we have a programme for every goal.

Each programme has a workout, diet plan and nutritious and delicious recipes that will really rev up your metabolism as well as encourage your body to lose fat and eliminate toxins, so you'll feel as good as you look. We also share our top tips for maximising and maintaining your results from page 17, from the best foods to munch to the kit you'll need.

Ready to transform your body? Take our quiz on page 10 to discover which plan will suit you, then turn to page 14 to work out your stats... And get started!

Have fun!

Joanna

WARNING: THESE PLANS WORK!

Contents

It's fast, furious and results-driven

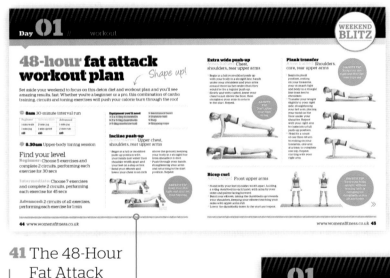

Ideal if time is short

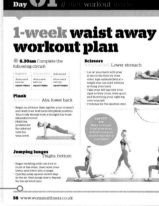

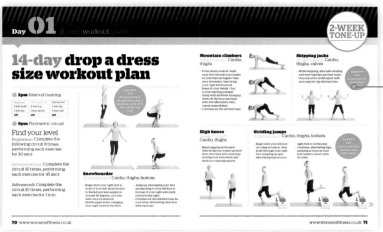

Perfect for the year's big events

WORKOUT BUDDY
Each plan comes with step-by-step instructions

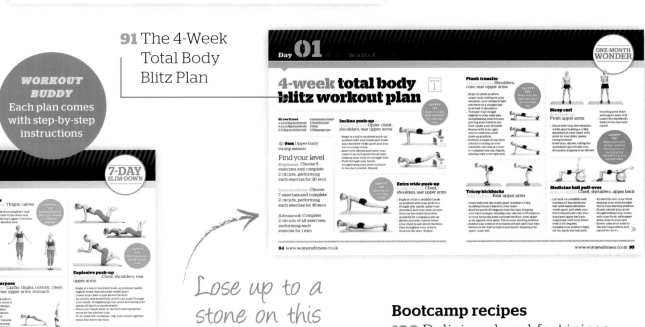

Lose up to a stone on this month-long plan

Bootcamp recipes

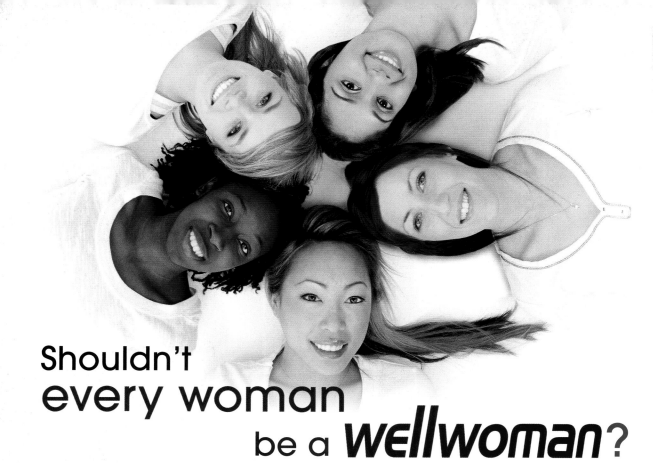

Shouldn't every woman be a *wellwoman*?

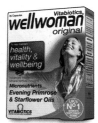 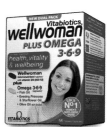 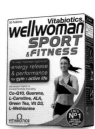 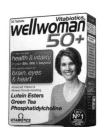 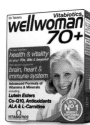 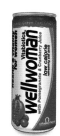

The UK's No. 1 supplements for women's health

Whether you are looking to support all-round vitality, sport and fitness, or maintain health over 50 and beyond, the **award winning Vitabiotics Wellwoman® range** offers **sensible, balanced formulae**. With 40 years experience, there's no women's supplement range more relied on than Vitabiotics.

Wellwoman supports

Originally developed with

Prof. A. H. Beckett[†]
OBE, PhD, DSc
Professor Emeritus,
University of London

From , Superdrug, Holland & Barrett,
Lloydspharmacy, GNC, supermarkets, health stores,
independent pharmacies & **www.vitabiotics.com**

Britain's leading supplements
for specific life stages

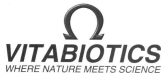

VITABIOTICS
WHERE NATURE MEETS SCIENCE

ADWEMMIXCONP 22-03-12

Get
started

Find the perfect plan for your goal, discover the secrets to success, then get to work!

Find your ultimate bootcamp plan

Want to be slimmer, stronger or more sculpted? Take our quiz and discover the perfect strategy for your goals

Whether you're after an instant slim-down or sustained weight loss, following the right diet and training is key. Take our quick quiz to find the bootcamp plan that will help you achieve the results you want. Simply answer each question as honestly as possible, tally your score and check the results opposite to find out which plan is your perfect fit.

What's your end goal?
A A flat tum in a bikini
B A looser waistband in your favourite jeans
C A more toned body
D To be stronger and lighter

What's your biggest challenge when it comes to weight loss?
A Lack of time
B Staying motivated
C Being inspired to cook healthy meals
D Avoiding a weight-loss plateau

The phrase which best describes your personality is:
A Impulsive and carefree
B Upbeat with a love for diversity in life
C Logical and driven
D Organised and consistent

Your mantra in life is:
A Time flies when you're having fun!
B Variety is the spice of life
C No pain, no gain
D You have to put the effort in to reap the rewards

What cheers you up after a bad day?
A An impromptu shopping spree
B A box of chocolates
C Dinner with your friends
D A big hug

For a diet to work for me it has to:
A Offer relatively quick results
B Work around my busy schedule
C Incorporate step-by-step recipes so I don't fall off the wagon
D Be healthy and sustainable

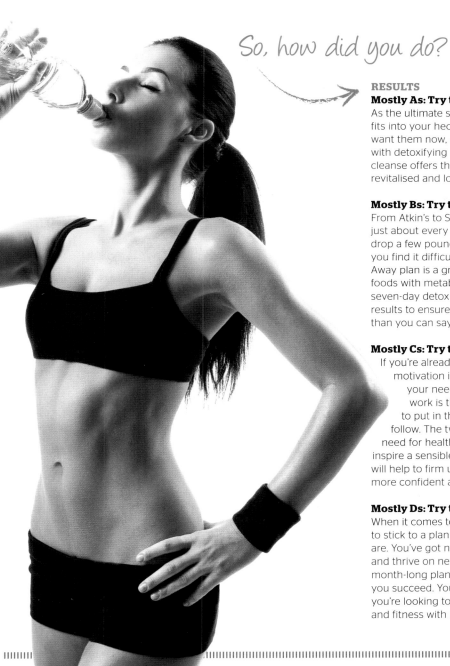

So, how did you do?

RESULTS

Mostly As: Try the 48-Hour Fat Attack Plan

As the ultimate social butterfly you need a plan that fits into your hectic schedule. You want results and you want them now, so this weekend blitz is ideal. Packed with detoxifying meals and fun workouts, this two-day cleanse offers the overhaul you need to ensure you feel revitalised and look ravishing in record time.

Mostly Bs: Try the 1-Week Waist Away Plan

From Atkin's to South Beach, you've tried and tested just about every diet on the market in the quest to drop a few pounds, but your fun-loving nature means you find it difficult to stay focused. The 1-Week Waist Away plan is a great solution. Combining cleansing foods with metabolism-boosting exercise plans, this seven-day detox offers quick, yet sensible weight-loss results to ensure you look leaner and feel lighter quicker than you can say 'flat tummy'.

Mostly Cs: Try the 14-Day Drop A Dress Size Plan

If you're already on the road to weight loss but your motivation is starting to wane, this plan will suit your needs. You're realistic and realise that hard work is the key to success, so you're prepared to put in the effort if you have a proper regime to follow. The two-week plan offers the guidance you need for healthy weight loss. The recipes will help inspire a sensible attitude to eating while the workouts will help to firm up trouble zones, leaving you feeling more confident and looking fab.

Mostly Ds: Try the 4-Week Total Body Blitz Plan

When it comes to shifting the pounds, you're most likely to stick to a plan that's as precise and organised as you are. You've got no problem following a strict regime and thrive on new challenges so you'll embark on the month-long plan with a positive outlook that will help you succeed. You're not a fan of fad diets – instead, you're looking to kick-start a healthy attitude to diet and fitness with results that can be sustained. ◼

10 rules
for weight-loss
success

Keep focused and achieve the body you've always wanted!

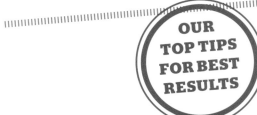

OUR TOP TIPS FOR BEST RESULTS

Embarking on a new diet and fitness routine can be daunting, but developing the right mindset will motivate you to reach your goals. Follow our essential guide to keeping your new healthy lifestyle on track...

1. Monitor your measurements

Muscle weighs more than fat, so ditch daily weigh-ins and monitor changes with a measuring tape instead. Take your measurements once a week and record your results as a reminder of your progress. See page 14 for advice on how to get the most from your measurements.

2. Create a schedule

Following a plan or writing down your diet and workout schedule week by week is vital for successful slimming. From meal planning to deciding when and where to work out, precise forward planning will help you stay on the bootcamp wagon.

3. Be patient

Small, subtle changes equal long-term success, so ease your way into your diet and fitness routine rather than jumping in with high hopes of losing a stone in a week. This way you'll be more likely to keep the weight off for good.

4. Enlist a bootcamp buddy

Getting a like-minded friend to join you in your new healthy lifestyle can make all the difference to your morale. Plan supermarket shopping trips together, invite each other over for homemade meals and phone each other when chocolate cravings strike!

5. Go shopping

Investing in flattering workout gear helps you to feel good about yourself. Hit the high street for tummy control tops, leg-lengthening capris and a snug sports bra to ensure you look and feel the part.

6. Treat yourself

Reward yourself – go on, you deserve it! Set yourself weekly targets, and when you reach them, shout yourself a pretty lipstick, a pair of shoes or a whole new outfit if you're feeling flash.

7. Challenge yourself

Whether it's being fit enough to run your first 5K or getting down to a size 10 in time for your best friend's wedding, having a goal to strive for is a great way to keep focused. Referring back to your end target will help when motivation slumps.

8. Keep active

To push your body into fat-burning mode, keep active throughout the day. Take the stairs instead of the lift, cycle or walk to work instead of taking the bus and do the housework with plenty of extra vigour!

9. Don't give up

It's normal to have off days, and one bad day isn't going to undo all your hard work. So don't beat yourself up if you've missed a fitness session or gorged on a takeaway – simply pick up where you left off tomorrow.

10. Stay motivated

Think of a time you felt good about yourself. That summer holiday where you were tanned and slim? Your 25th birthday? Stick up a photo of the 'old' you as a constant reminder of what you want to achieve. 🆆

Measure up

Don't just rely on the scales – uncover your
true results by tracking your inch loss

>> Because all of our bootcamp plans combine
fat-blasting interval cardio sessions, toning
exercises and a diet plan, you won't just lose
weight on the scales, you'll feel and look slimmer,
lighter and tighter all over.

Plus, it's important to note that what the scales
say can be misleading as your body builds muscle
mass. So, make sure you know your body and its
measurements to see real results.

Use the guide here to measure your stats so you
can track your progress, whatever plan you embark
on. Make sure you take your body measurements in
the same places each time for accurate results.

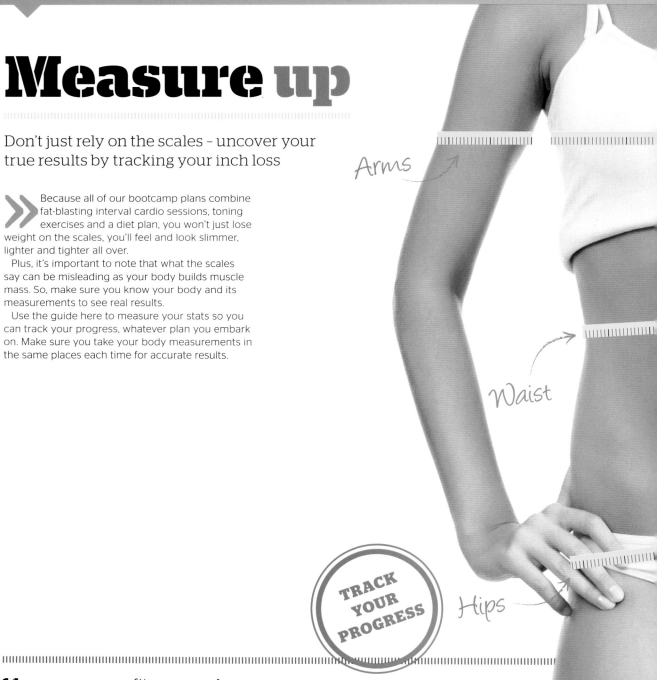

Arms

Waist

TRACK
YOUR
PROGRESS

Hips

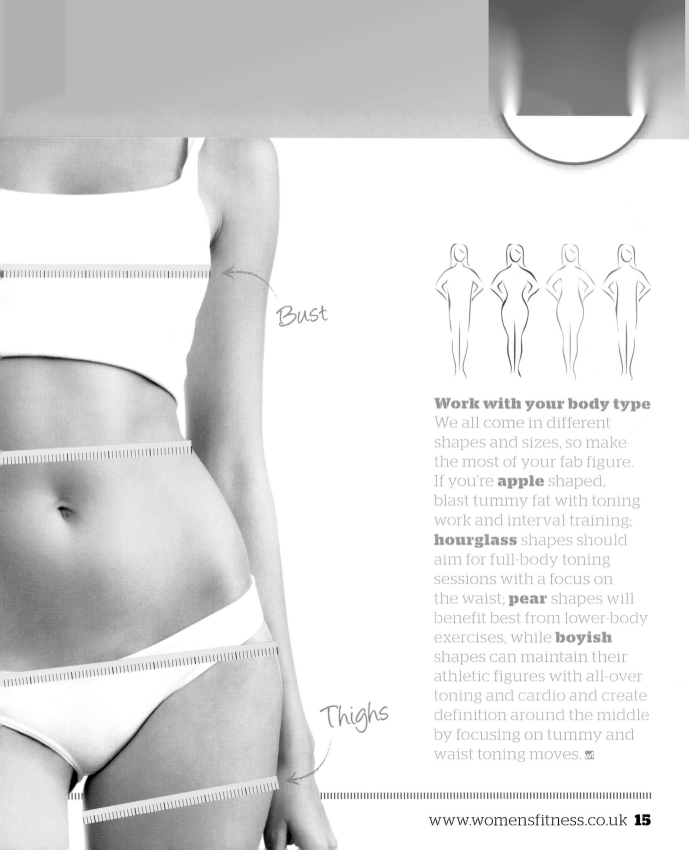

Bust

Thighs

Work with your body type

We all come in different shapes and sizes, so make the most of your fab figure. If you're **apple** shaped, blast tummy fat with toning work and interval training; **hourglass** shapes should aim for full-body toning sessions with a focus on the waist; **pear** shapes will benefit best from lower-body exercises, while **boyish** shapes can maintain their athletic figures with all-over toning and cardio and create definition around the middle by focusing on tummy and waist toning moves. 🔟

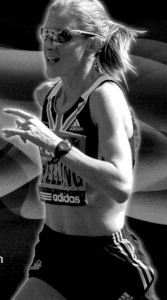
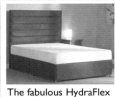
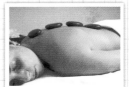
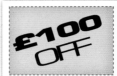
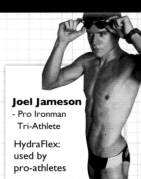
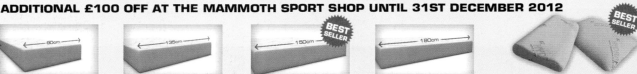

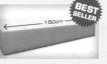
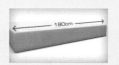

shape up

Find out how to get the best
from your workouts and really
maximise your results

Your workout
questions ...*Answered*

Get the most out of your bootcamp
sessions with this need-to-know advice

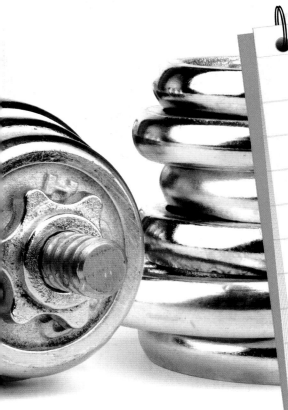

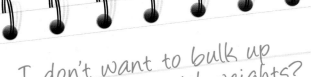

*I don't want to bulk up
– should I avoid weights?*

It's a huge myth that you'll look like Arnold
Schwarzenegger once you start picking up
the dumbbells. Someone with incredibly
huge muscles needs to follow a strict,
regimented diet and weights routine for
months to develop and maintain that kind
of physique, so it isn't easy. Doing weights
will, however, really boost your metabolism
and in turn burn fat, so don't be scared
of them! Stick to low reps of the heaviest
weights you can manage safely if you're
really worried about putting on muscle,
as it's the higher repetitions that are more
likely to build your muscle size.

I go to the gym regularly but still can't see a difference. What am I doing wrong? If you're the kind of gym bunny who turns up without a plan and simply uses whatever machines are free, you might wonder why your longed-for results are failing to appear. Every fitness regime needs a proper structure. Think of it this way: if your goal is flexibility, would you do a spinning class? Probably not. Consistency is key, so define your goal, whether it's weight loss, strength or fitness, and use your workouts to target this for six to eight weeks. Then, change it up so your body doesn't become complacent and your results continue to progress.

'Use your workouts to target a goal for six to eight weeks'

Why do I need to pay attention to my heart rate?

Knowing your heart rate is useful for lots of reasons. Your resting heart rate (how many times your heart beats per minute at rest) is a good indicator of how fit you are. You can monitor your fitness by checking this regularly. The lower it is, the fitter you are. Paying attention to your heart rate while exercising lets you know how much effort you're putting in, too, by comparing it to your maximum heart rate (women can calculate their MHR by multiplying their age by 0.64 and subtracting the answer from 211). This is particularly useful when interval training: during the sprint periods, you can check that you're working hard enough, and during the rest intervals, you can monitor your heart rate slowing back down before you launch into another sprint session. »

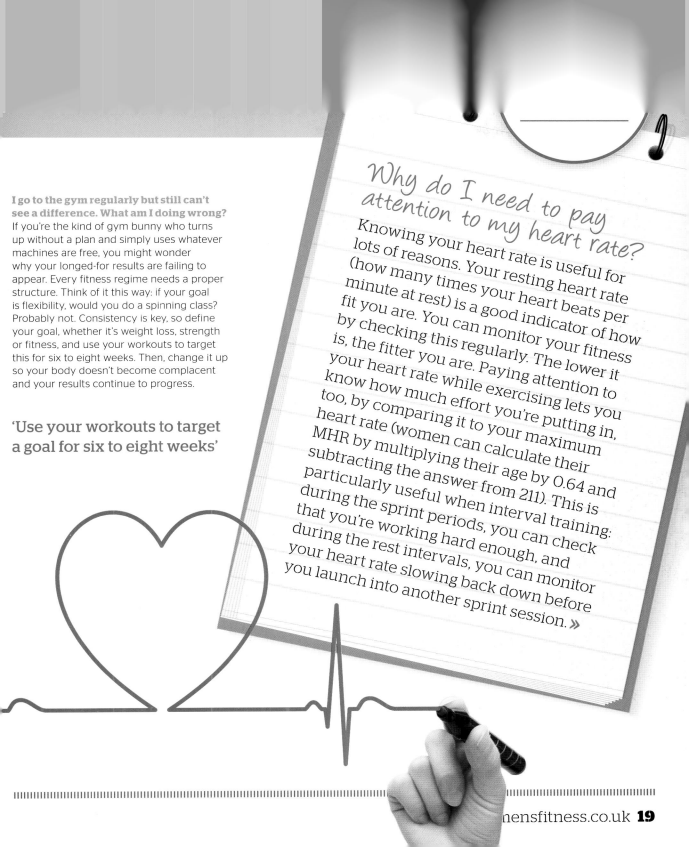

I'm new to exercise and worried I might injure myself. How do you recommend starting exercise?
If you're completely new to exercise, your muscles need to get used to the movements you're likely to be performing in a workout. You can do this by using resistance machines, which will safely guide your muscles through a range of movement with control and stability. Make sure you start with light resistance just to practise the motion. Once you feel comfortable though, move onto free weights. These are much more beneficial as they work your balance, coordination and stability muscles, too, making the movements far more functional and useful to you in everyday life.

'You won't see the results of your hard work if there is fat hiding the muscle'

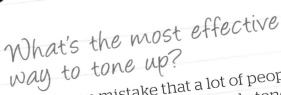

What's the most effective way to tone up?

A common mistake that a lot of people make is to work towards muscle tone by doing hundreds of exercises targeted at a particular problem area, but you won't see the results of your hard work if there is still fat hiding the muscle. You can't turn fat into muscle, or vice versa, but you can get rid of the fat that lies on top of the muscle. Lots of high-repetition exercises won't do this, though, and will only build the muscle underneath the fat, so unless you want to keep your toned tummy, honed thighs and pert bum under wraps, you need to trim the fat by performing plenty of metabolism-boosting workouts that will get your calorie-burn sky high. Think high-resistance, low-repetition free weights routines and intense cardio, such as interval training. wf

FOCUS ON YOUR GOALS. NOT YOUR FEET.

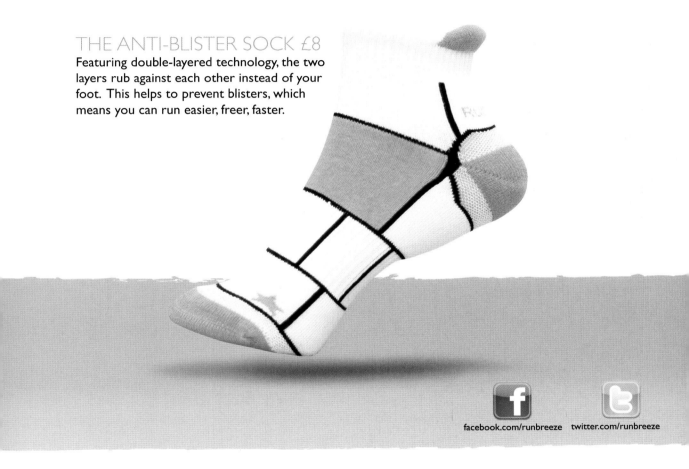

THE ANTI-BLISTER SOCK £8

Featuring double-layered technology, the two layers rub against each other instead of your foot. This helps to prevent blisters, which means you can run easier, freer, faster.

facebook.com/runbreeze   twitter.com/runbreeze

Supercharge your workouts

Want to make sure that every minute you spend working out *really* counts? Follow these top tips to get on the fast track to fitness

Try intervals

Whether you're running, rowing or doing a resistance workout, make sure you adopt interval training. This means working at a very high intensity, followed by a period of rest to allow you to return right back to the high intensity, and so on. This type of start-and-stop style training really puts your muscles under strain (in a good way!), which will in turn give your metabolism a real boost, so it keeps burning fat long after your workout is over. Score!

Drink up

We all know it's vital to stay hydrated, whether you're exercising or not, but if you're working out it's essential to up your intake accordingly. Aim for an extra 500ml per hour of exercise you're doing, and don't just drink up during your workout – it's important to be properly hydrated before you start and after you've finished, too. It might be tempting to reach for a sugar hit from energy drinks, tablets or gels, but you don't want to undo all that hard work in the gym. The sugar content in these are high, so unless you're doing an endurance workout that lasts more than two hours, stick with good old water.

Ladies should lift

There was a time when us girls would stick to the cross-trainers and leave the free weights areas to the men, but no longer! Lots of women are still dubious about using weights in fear of building up a scary Hulk-esque physique, but unless you're specifically training towards this with a bespoke diet and regimented workouts, you've got nothing to worry about. Rather, weights can help you to burn fat without losing definition, have a faster metabolism and make you stronger. Who wouldn't want that? Incorporate dumbbells, weighted bars and more into your workouts for a sculpted figure. ▥

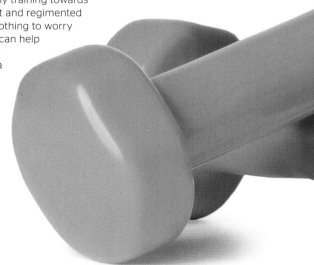

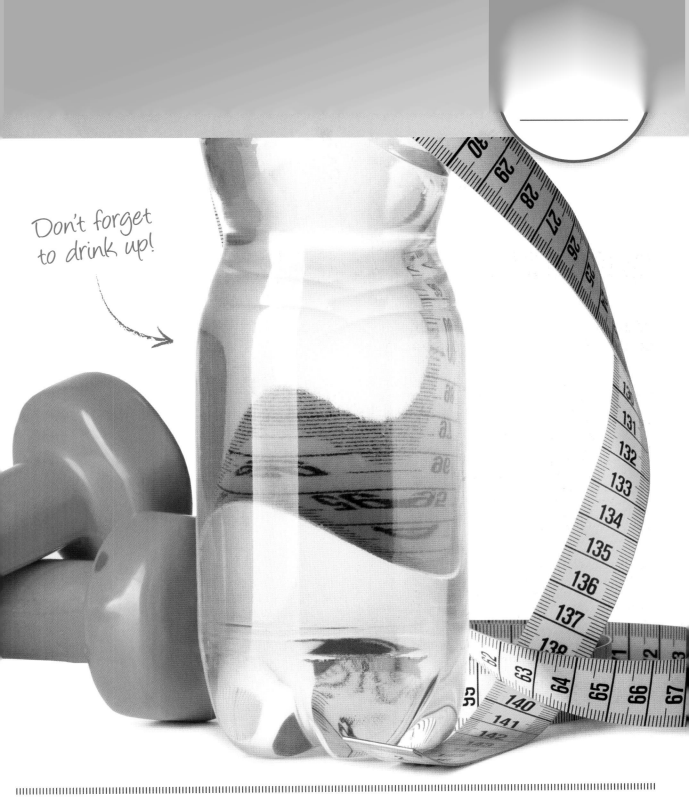

Don't forget to drink up!

CHΔNGE

YOUR REFLECTION

s arguably the most sophisticated diet
available today. Reflex Nutrition have used
nces in protein and weight loss science to
oduct that's specifically designed to help
healthy, well defined and toned body.

There are many surveys published analyzing the
CLA (conjugated linoleic acid) content of foods from
around the world which show that intake of CLA is
lower than in scientific studies where beneficial health
effects are induced.

Research also suggests that in order to obtain the
reported health benefits of CLA, supplementation
is required.

Reflex Diet Protein™ is the only sports supplement
available today that uses a 3.2g daily dose of
CLA which is substantiated as an effective dose
by research.

Each serving of Reflex Diet Protein™ is packed with
additional diet support. Green Tea extract is added for
its long standing reputation for aiding dieters.

Diet Protein™ contains no added sugar or maltodextrin.
It's perfect for dieters wanting to restrict their
carbohydrate content.

Diet Protein™ comes in a variety of mouthwatering
flavours, all of which have been up against a taste
test panel to ensure that they are the best tasting
diet shakes on the market.

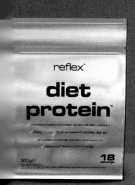

RRP £32.99

00g - 18 x 50g servings

about our products at:

x-nutrition.com

it & join our Facebook
eflex Nutrition Ltd

 @ReflexNutrition

ecotricity

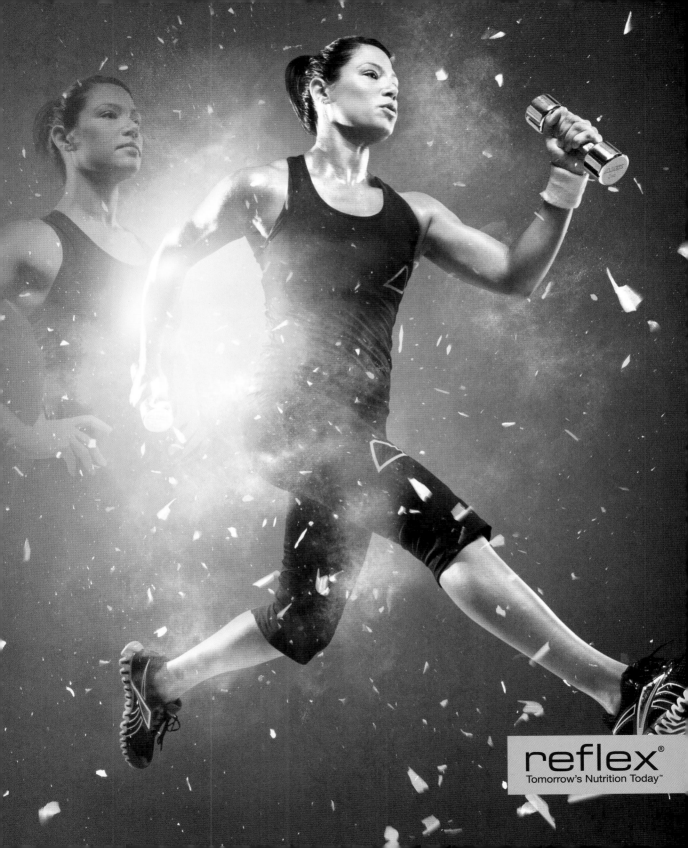

Essential kit

Great gear will help you look and feel the part

Go for bold in bright leggings

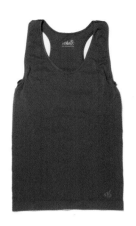

Stand out as you work out in a bright top. This No Balls seamless tank has an inbuilt bra for real comfort and support – stock up with a rainbow of colours.
» **£27, www.noballs.co.uk**

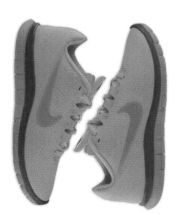

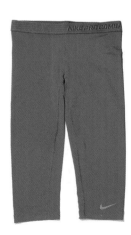

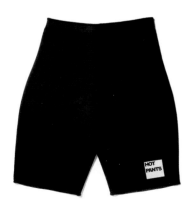

These Nike Women Free Advantage trainers are perfect if you really want to *feel* your run! They offer premium support in a stylish, lightweight shoe.
» **£80, www.nikestore.com**

Make a real impact at the gym in Nike's Pro Core capri tights. They use Dri-Fit fabric to keep you cool and comfortable while looking hot.
» **£30, www.nikestore.com**

Supercharge your workouts with pants that help you burn more cals! Zaggora HotPants are a clever way to really rev up your energy expenditure.
» **£44.99, www.zaggora.com**

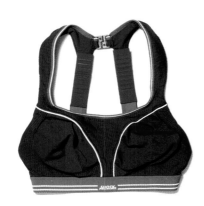

A good sports bra is a must for every workout. We love the patriotic look and supportive feel of this Shock Absorber Ultimate Run Bra.
» **£37, www.shockabsorber.co.uk**

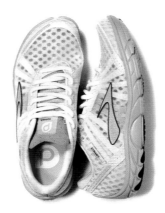

Make sure your feet are well supported while you run, sprint and jog – it'll make all the difference. These Brooks Pure Connect trainers fit the bill.
» **£90, www.brooksrunning.co.uk**

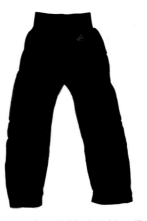

Three-quarter length black tights will be a staple of your workout wardrobe. Invest in these seamless No Balls leggings for a flattering fit.
» **£29, www.noballs.co.uk**

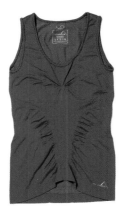

This Striders Edge Engineered Climate Map vest is designed to keep you cool and dry while you're on the move, and the ruching masks trouble spots, too.
» **£55, www.stridersedge.com**

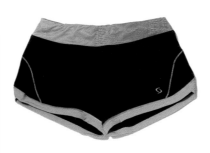

Feeling confident? Rock your newly honed and toned legs in these cute and colourful running shorts from Moving Comfort.
» **£29, www.movingcomfort.co.uk**

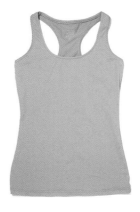

Brighten up grey days in this Athlete racer-back vest from Sweaty Betty. The bright hue is bound to put a spring in your step!
» **£28, www.sweatybetty.com**

Must-have gear

Invest in this equipment for endless workout options

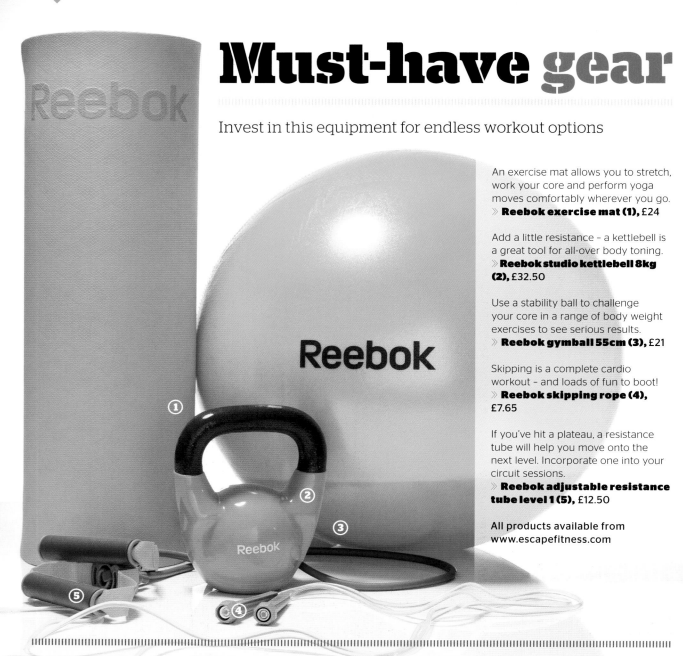

An exercise mat allows you to stretch, work your core and perform yoga moves comfortably wherever you go.
» **Reebok exercise mat (1),** £24

Add a little resistance – a kettlebell is a great tool for all-over body toning.
» **Reebok studio kettlebell 8kg (2),** £32.50

Use a stability ball to challenge your core in a range of body weight exercises to see serious results.
» **Reebok gymball 55cm (3),** £21

Skipping is a complete cardio workout – and loads of fun to boot!
» **Reebok skipping rope (4),** £7.65

If you've hit a plateau, a resistance tube will help you move onto the next level. Incorporate one into your circuit sessions.
» **Reebok adjustable resistance tube level 1 (5),** £12.50

All products available from www.escapefitness.com

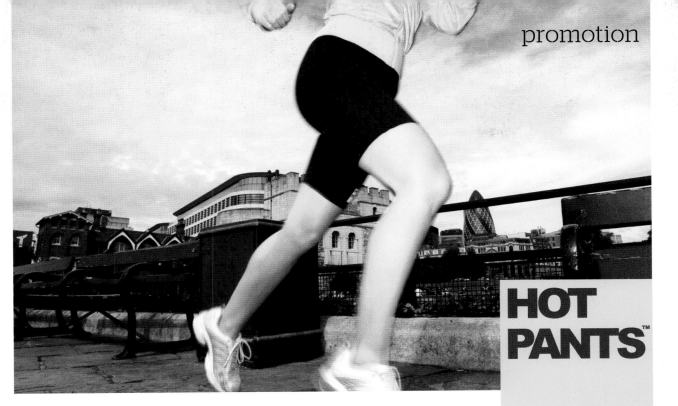

HOT PANTS™

Hot stuff

Want to shape up for summer? Supercharge your weight loss with Zaggora HotPants

Now that the weather's warmer, summer's skimpy shorts and skirts are great motivation for toning up and getting in shape! But, before you hit the gym, invest in a pair of Zaggora HotPants, which claim to help you burn calories four times faster, increasing the effectiveness of any exercise.

Already a global weight-loss phenomenon, Zaggora HotPants work by stimulating your natural body heat to raise your core temperature. The extra heat increases your energy expenditure during exercise. Wear them at the gym to boost your workout or under your everyday clothes to help you tone up on the go.

Zaggora HotPants are the brainchild of UK-based Dessi Bell, who came up with the idea in the lead up to her wedding when she wanted to look her best. Since their launch in 2011, more than 400,000 pairs of Zaggora HotPants have been sold to women in 110 countries. They've also been a hit on the celebrity scene – reportedly, Holly Willoughby, Tess Daly and Holly Valance are all avid fans!

Buy a pair of Zaggora HotPants today and reap the benefits all summer long. For more information and to shop, log on to zaggora.com.

 Visit www.facebook.com/zaggora to see the positive feedback from thousands of real women

 Follow Zaggora HotPants on Twitter @zaggora

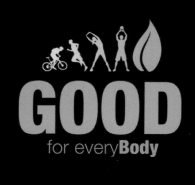
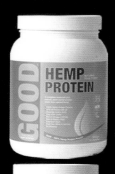

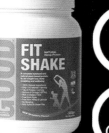

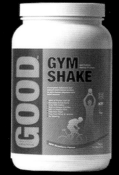

Smart eating

These savvy food tips will help you shape your dream figure

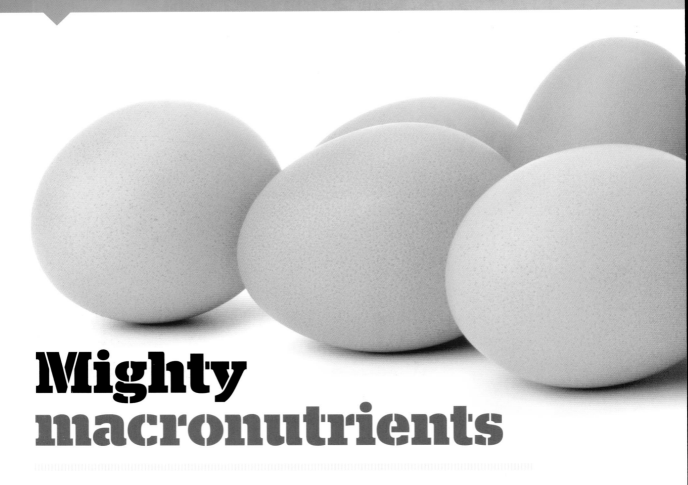

Mighty macronutrients

Pile your plate with the right food groups to keep weight off for good

Want to fight hunger pangs, stubborn cravings and best of all, shift your excess pounds forever? Then make sure your diet is up to scratch. Macronutrients, a food group encompassing protein, carbohydrates and fats, provide the foundation of good nutrition, helping to keep your waistline in check for the long haul. These foods fuel your body with energy and nutrients to support growth and repair, and help to regulate your body's functions.

PROTEIN

Protein plays an essential role in any healthy diet. This growth-and-repair nutrient provides the building blocks of muscle, skin and blood. It helps to keep your immune system working efficiently, maintains healthy skin, hair and nails and keeps you feeling fuller for longer, so it's important to make sure you're getting enough in your diet. As a minimum guide you need 8g of protein per kilogram of

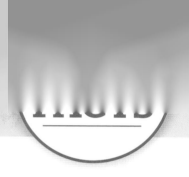

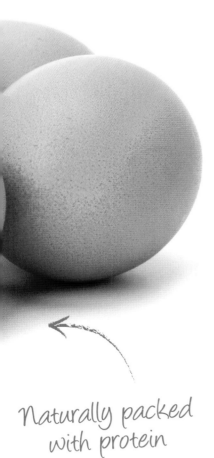

Naturally packed with protein

> '**These foods fuel your body with energy and nutrients to support growth and repair**'

high levels of saturated fat. Protein from plant sources helps lower cholesterol and contains a broad spectrum of nutrients, too.

CARBOHYDRATES

There are two groups of carbohydrates – simple carbohydrates, such as those found in white bread, pasta, refined cakes and biscuits; and complex carbohydrates, found in wholegrain pasta, brown rice and wholemeal bread, which form the brain's primary energy source to fuel your muscles. Simple carbohydrates release sugar into the bloodstream quickly, causing a sharp spike in blood sugar levels followed by an abrupt dip. This results in a lull in energy, and can cause sugar cravings and mood swings. Complex carbohydrates, on the other hand, help your body sustain more balanced blood sugar levels as they take longer for the body to digest, so they help to keep your energy levels raised for a longer amount of time.

FATS

It might surprise you to hear that to lose fat you have to eat fat, but it's true! The right kind of fats, known as essential fatty acids (EFAs), help to boost metabolism, aid brain and nerve function, balance hormones and even improve your skin, hair and nails. There are three types of EFAs: omega-3, 6 and 9. It's important to get the ratio correct. Most of us eat

enough omega-6 and too much omega-9, but not enough omega-3, which is full of amazing anti-inflammatory properties. To boost your intake of healthy omega-3 fats, include food such as oily fish (think salmon, mackerel and herring), and plenty of raw nuts and seeds in your daily diet. To maintain a healthy diet and avoid putting on weight, take care to avoid trans fats (found in processed food such as cakes, biscuits and ready meals) and only eat saturated fats such as those found in butter and red meat in moderation. 🖬

The perfect plate
Half of your plate should be made up of vegetables (dark green leafy veg plus a selection of brightly coloured veg) and the other half should be made up of one quarter protein, one eighth complex carbohydrates and one eighth good fats.

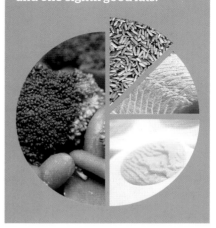

body weight, however if you're exercising you'll need to increase your intake. Good sources of protein include lean meat, poultry, eggs, lentils, beans, nuts, seeds, soya and cheese. It's best to include a mix of protein sources in your diet. Animal sources contain a more absorbable form of protein, however they often contain

Maximise your metabolism

Rev up your body's natural fat furnace with these clever tips

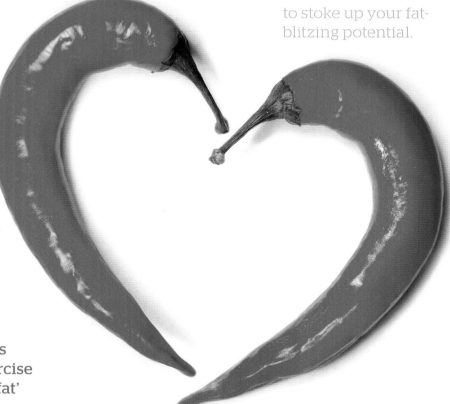

>> Believe it or not, you can trick your body into melting away the pounds simply by boosting your basal metabolic rate – the calories your body burns at rest.

A number of factors, from your fitness regime to your diet choices, genetics and lifestyle, influence the effectiveness of your metabolism – and while you can't change your genes, you can take certain steps to help speed up your body's natural energy regulator.

Missing meals, skipping the gym and eating a nutrient-deficient diet will all slow your metabolism down. Instead, follow our simple tips to help rewire your metabolic rate and ramp up your weight loss. It's simple!

Spice up your plate
Research suggests that hot spices such as chilli raise the metabolism for up to three hours after eating. Add chopped fresh chilli to soups, stews and curries to stoke up your fat-blitzing potential.

'A decent night's sleep is as important as diet and exercise when it comes to melting fat'

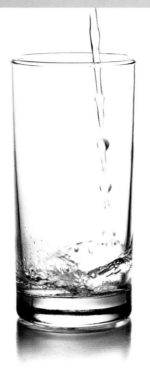
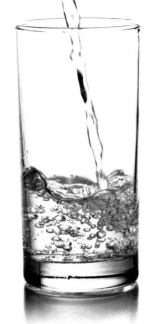
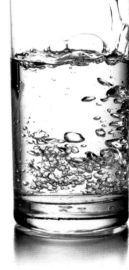

'You can take certain steps to help speed up your body's natural energy regulator'

Eat a good breakfast

Skipping breakfast causes your body to plummet into starvation mode and retain fat as it naturally clings onto energy stores when food is scarce. Start the day with a nutritious meal: a breakfast such as oats with nuts, seeds and a handful of berries will keep you full for hours.

Switch off the heating

Your body expends energy to help regulate its temperature, so when you're a little cold your body is forced to burn more energy to generate heat.

Mix up your workouts

Variety is the spice of life – and this applies to your workouts, too. Keep your sessions short and sharp, stepping up the intensity with interval training (alternating sprints with slower-paced exercise) in favour of exercising at a steady pace. This will boost your metabolism and increase the amount of calories your body burns at rest.

Love your lymphatic system

Boosting the function of your lymphatic system is key to keeping your body healthy. This important system removes excess fluid and metabolic waste from your body. Lymph fluid flows upwards from your feet, passing through special filtration points called lymph nodes where toxins are eliminated. Daily dry body brushing before showering helps to improve this process. Start at your feet and move upwards, using gentle strokes.

Hydrate with H$_2$O

Guzzling back two litres of water a day is an easy way to whittle down your waistline with minimum effort required! Research shows that drinking chilled water has added body-boosting benefits. How does it work? Sipping on ice-cold water raises your metabolism as the body has to burn calories bringing the water to body temperature. Easy peasy!

Sleep tight

A decent night's sleep is as important as a good diet and exercise when it comes to melting fat. Sleep deprivation lowers the metabolism and throws the body's appetite-regulating hormones, leptin and ghrelin, off balance. Try to lull your body into a sleepy state with a hot bath and chamomile tea, and take care not to exercise, work or watch TV too late at night, as these activities stimulate the mind when it needs to power down. »

Get supplement savvy

Magnesium
Struggling to control your chocolate cravings? You may be low in magnesium. This mineral naturally balances hormones and helps to improve exercise performance. Try Floradix Magnesium (1), £8.33, www.victoriahealth.com.

Conjugated Linoleic Acid (CLA)
CLA is a fatty acid with potent antioxidant powers. It helps to decrease absorption of fat and sugar into fat cells and improves blood sugar balance. Try Nature's Plus Mega CLA (2), £32.80, www.nutricentre.com.

Chromium
This weight-controlling mineral plays an important role in regulating the actions of the blood sugar-balancing hormone insulin. Supplement with the picolinate form, as it's easily absorbed. Try BioCare Nutrisorb Chromium (3), £17, www.biocare.co.uk.

Omega-3
Essential fatty acids (EFAs), notably omega-3, help you lose weight by increasing the enzymes needed for your body to burn fat. Studies also indicate supplementation of EFAs combined with exercise helps to further enhance the fat-burning benefits. Try Vitabiotics Ultra Omega-3 High Potency (4), £10.15, www.vitabiotics.com.

Alpha Lipoic Acid (ALA)
This powerful antioxidant speeds up the body's fat-burning processes by enhancing the body's ability to break down food for energy. Plus, it helps to regulate sensitivity to insulin. Try Solgar Alpha Lipoic Acid (5), £19.95, www.revital.com.

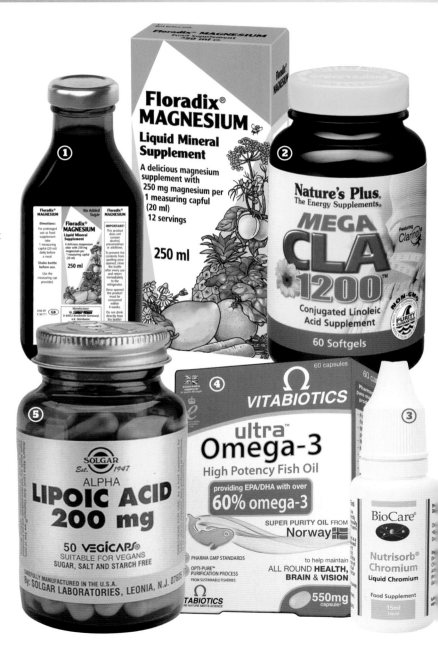

Flat-belly foods

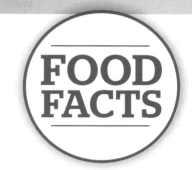

FOOD FACTS

Whittle down your middle with these tummy-friendly treats

>> Our tummies are the first place to show the signs of weight gain and, frustratingly, one of the hardest areas to shift fat from. Salt, processed food and sugar can all cause the body to retain fluid, leading to uncomfortable bloating. Fortunately, munching the right foods can knock inches off your middle by eliminating excess water and revving up your metabolism. Try these eight tummy-friendly foods for a flatter stomach.

Oats

A steaming bowl of porridge is a filling source of complex carbohydrates and fibre. Oats also contain a substance called mucilage, which supports and soothes the digestive tract.

Natural yoghurt

Yoghurt contains friendly bacteria which promotes good intestinal health and banishes uncomfortable bloating symptoms. Avoid sweetened yoghurts and load up on natural Greek yoghurt instead.

Nettle tea

It's not exactly a food, but it should be on your shopping list. Nettle tea acts as a diuretic which means it helps to reduce water retention. Nettle is also anti-inflammatory and packed with nutrients. Drink at least two cups a day to tame your tummy.

Papaya

Go exotic! Research shows that the enzyme papain which is found in papaya helps to aid digestion. Try adding it to a fruit salad or serve it with yoghurt to help beat the bloat.

Leafy greens

Load up your plate with leafy greens such as spinach, kale and broccoli. These nutrient-dense veggies help aid detoxification and clear out waste products. »

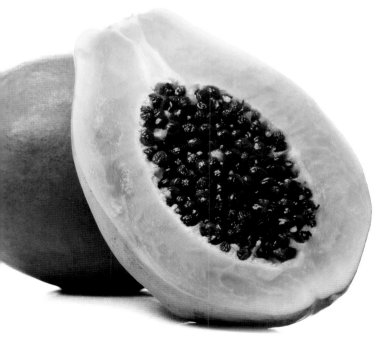

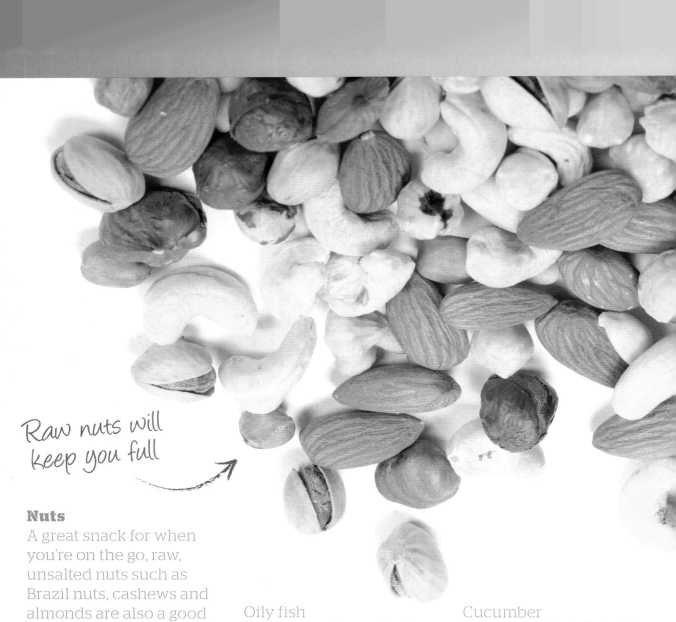

Raw nuts will keep you full

Nuts

A great snack for when you're on the go, raw, unsalted nuts such as Brazil nuts, cashews and almonds are also a good source of omega-3 fatty acids, which help to blast belly fat. Aim for a few small handfuls every day.

Oily fish

Oily fish such as salmon, mackerel, anchovies, sardines and herring are packed with omega-3 fatty acids which help to keep your waistline trim by revving up your metabolism. They're also great for your heart and brain.

Cucumber

This salad staple helps to flush out toxins through its diuretic actions. It's a high-water food, which means you can eat loads without worrying about calories. Serve it as a snack with houmous or add a few slices to water for a tasty twist. ⬛

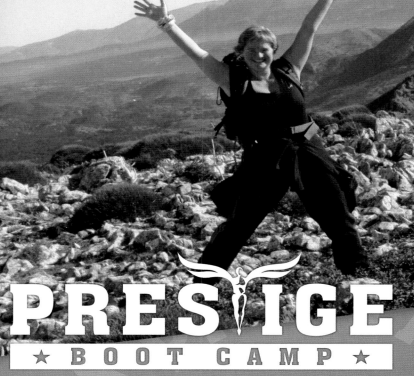
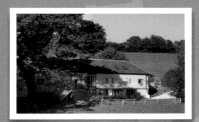
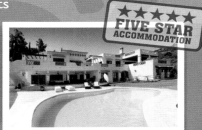

Eat a rainbow

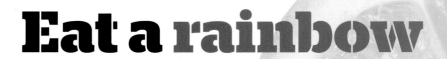

Colour-code your plate for the ultimate health boost

Antioxidants are the ultimate health-givers when it comes to food. These naturally occurring chemicals which give fruit and veg their bright hues help to fend off the signs of ageing and fight disease. They work by helping to counteract the effect of free radicals – the baddies of the food world. Free radicals are unstable molecules that negatively alter the structure of your body's cells and contribute to a range of health conditions and diseases. To boost your body's health, chow down on around seven or nine portions of brightly coloured fruit and vegetables every day.

'Antioxidants help to fend off the signs of ageing and fight disease'

Red
Lycopene is an antioxidant with healing powers. Thought to help prevent cancer, this edible chemical is found in tomatoes, strawberries, peppers and radishes, and has increased benefits when cooked.

Green
Dark green vegetables serve as a fantastic source of the antioxidants lutein and zeaxanthin, which both work to preserve eyesight and fight off cancer. Munch on spinach, watercress, rocket, asparagus, avocado and kale for your hit.

Purple and blue
Packed with amazing antioxidants, purple and blue fruit and vegetables contain health-promoting chemicals called anthocyanins. These help to keep your heart functioning properly, reduce the risk of age-related memory loss and may even help ward off urinary tract infections. Get your fill with plenty of blueberries, blackberries, plums and aubergines.

Orange and yellow
Orange and yellow foods such as carrots, sweet potatoes and oranges are full of antioxidants including vitamin C, beta-cryptoxanthin and beta-carotene (which converts to vitamin A). These goodies have a wealth of health benefits, from improving vision, boosting your skin health, strengthening the immune system and protecting the digestive tract lining.

48-hour
fat attack plan

This speedy shape-up gets results

You'll have to clear your diary for this but it is possible to slim down in just two days!

Be sure to fill in your vital statistics on page 54, so you can measure your results

Caution: As with any diet, you should consult your doctor before starting this plan and if you experience any unpleasant symptoms you should stop the diet and see a healthcare professional immediately. This plan is not suitable for those who are underweight, pregnant or planning on becoming pregnant, or breastfeeding. This plan should not be followed for more than 48 hours.

Things to remember

The weekend blitz is fast and furious, so follow these rules closely to achieve the best results

Equipment you'll need
» Juicer to juice fruit and vegetables
» Blender or hand blender for soups

» Our fast detox diet plan is designed to get you feeling and looking lighter and trimmer, especially around that all-important tummy area, in just one weekend. Your menu consists of juices and soups, plus some nuts and seeds and fruit to snack on. It may sound radical, but it's designed to be followed for no more than 48 hours.

The rules

» This plan consists of three 'meals' and three snacks per day. Breakfast is a juice; lunch and dinner are soups. The morning and afternoon snacks are both two tablespoons of mixed raw nuts and/or seeds and fruit. The day ends with an overnight detox drink, which is a light miso soup.

» Drink 1.5 litres of water a day.

» Take the following supplements every morning with your breakfast:
» Multivitamin/mineral
» Omega-3
» Mixed antioxidants

» Exercise and relax. Follow the exercise plan for each day and aim to sleep at least seven hours a night. You may also want to have a nap during the day.

» Don't drink coffee, tea, cola or other caffeinated drinks, including green tea. Replace them with water, or herbal teas and decaffeinated coffee without milk.

» Don't drink alcohol of any kind.

» Don't drink fruit juice, smoothies or fruit cordials. The only juices you should drink are those you have made according to the recipes on the plan.

» Don't eat any dairy products (milk, cheese, yoghurt); protein foods (meat, fish, eggs or vegetarian protein like tofu); fats (butter or oil); starchy carbs (bread, pasta, rice, potatoes, cakes and biscuits); or beans (lentils, chickpeas, kidney beans, etc).

» No chocolate!

48-hour fat attack diet plan

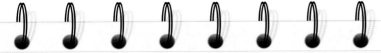

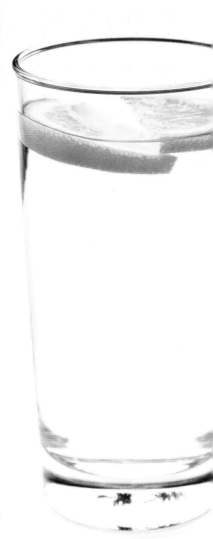

7am Lemon cleanse
» 1 glass of room-temperature water with a squeeze of lemon

7.30am Breakfast
» 1 beetroot liver cleanse juice (p120)
» Supplements

10.30am Snack
» 1 apple and 2 tablespoons of mixed raw nuts and/or seeds (Brazil nuts, almonds, walnuts and pumpkin or sunflower seeds)

1pm Lunch
» Green goddess soup (p122)

3.30pm Snack
» 2 tablespoons of mixed raw nuts and/or seeds and 2 handfuls of blueberries

7pm Dinner
» Cauliflower detox soup (p122)

10pm Overnight detox drink
» 1 cup of instant miso soup

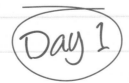

Day 1

48-hour fat attack workout plan

Shape up!

Set aside your weekend to focus on this detox diet and workout plan and you'll see amazing results, fast. Whether you're a beginner or a pro, this combination of cardio training, circuits and toning exercises will push your calorie burn through the roof

🕐 8am 30-minute interval run

Beginner	Intermediate	Advanced
1-min walk	2-min jog	1-min jog
1-min jog	1-min sprint	2-min run
x15	**x10**	**x10**

🕐 8.30am Upper-body toning session

Find your level

Beginner: Choose 5 exercises and complete 2 circuits, performing each exercise for 30 secs

Intermediate: Choose 7 exercises and complete 2 circuits, performing each exercise for 45 secs

Advanced: 2 circuits of all exercises, performing each exercise for 1 min

Equipment you'll need
» 2 x 4-8kg dumbbells
» 2 x 3-5kg dumbbells
» 5-8kg medicine ball
» Resistance band
» Stability ball
» Step
» Skipping rope

Incline push-up
Areas trained: Upper chest, shoulders, rear upper arms

» Begin in a full or modified push-up position with your hands just wider than shoulder-width apart and your feet on a step or box.
» Bend your elbows and lower your chest to an inch above the ground, keeping your body in a straight line from shoulders to feet.
» Push through your hands, straightening your arms and returning to the start position. Repeat.

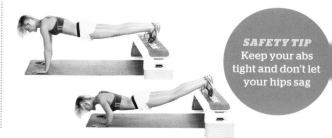

SAFETY TIP
Keep your abs tight and don't let your hips sag

Extra wide push-up
Areas trained: Chest, shoulders, rear upper arms

» Begin in a full or modified push-up with your body in a straight line, hands under your shoulders and your arms around three inches wider than they would be for a regular push-up.
» Slowly and with control, lower your chest to just above the floor, then straighten your arms to return to the start. Repeat.

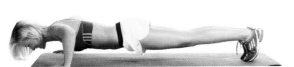

Plank transfer
Areas trained: Shoulders, core, rear upper arms

» Begin in plank position, resting on your forearms, your stomach tight and body in a straight line from feet to shoulders.
» Transfer your weight slightly to your right side, straightening your left arm, placing your hand on the floor under your shoulder. Repeat with your right arm to come into a full push-up position.
» Hold for a count of one then return to resting on your forearms, one arm at a time, to complete one rep. Repeat, starting with your right arm.

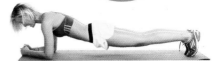
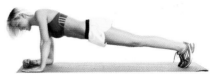
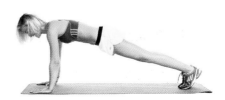

Bicep curl
Area trained: Front upper arms

» Stand with your feet shoulder-width apart, holding a 4-8kg dumbbell in each hand, with arms by your sides and palms facing forward.
» Bend your elbows, taking the dumbbells up towards your shoulders, keeping your elbows touching your sides with upper arms still.
» Lower the dumbbells down to the start and repeat.

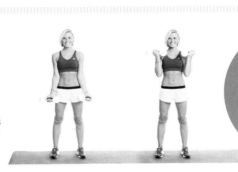

High row
Area trained:
Upper back

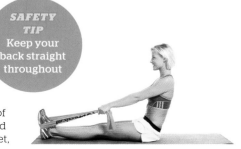

SAFETY TIP
Keep your back straight throughout

» Begin seated with your legs straight out in front of you and a resistance band wrapped around your feet, holding an end in each hand. There should be a little tension in the band at this point.

» Bring your hands towards your shoulders, taking your elbows up and out so they are level with your shoulders. Return to the start and repeat.

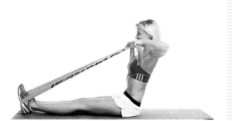

Medicine ball pull-over
Areas trained: Chest, shoulders, upper back

SAFETY TIP
Keep your tummy tight throughout

» Sit on a stability ball holding a 5-8kg medicine ball with hands shoulder-width apart, and walk your feet forward until only your head, neck and upper back are supported, with your knees bent at 90 degrees.

» Keeping your stomach tight, lift the medicine ball until it's directly over your chest, keeping your arms extended straight – this is your starting position.

» Slowly extend your arms straight behind you, in line with your body, with upper arms close to your ears.

» Slowly raise your arms to the starting position and repeat.

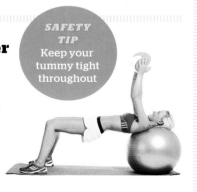

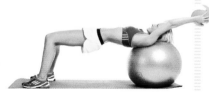

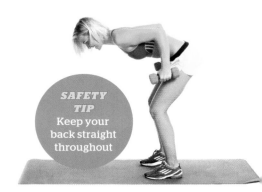

SAFETY TIP
Keep your back straight throughout

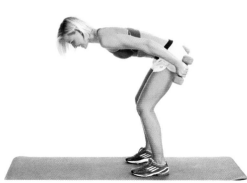

Tricep kickbacks
Area trained: Rear upper arms

» Stand with feet hip-width apart, holding a 3-5kg dumbbell in each hand by your sides.

» Bend forward 90 degrees from the hips, keeping your back straight, bending your elbows to 90 degrees so your forearms point towards the floor, your upper arms against your sides. This is your starting position.

» Slowly extend your elbows, so your hands are level with your hips.

» Return to the start and repeat, keeping your upper arms still.

Shadow boxing
Areas trained:
Shoulders, arms

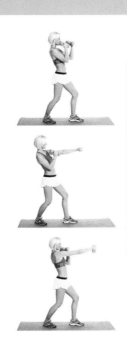

» Stand with your left foot slightly in front of your right and your left shoulder slightly in front of your right.
» Quickly punch straight ahead with your left hand, bringing it back and then repeating with your right hand. Continue for the allotted time.
» Hold a dumbbell in each hand to increase the difficulty if required.

SAFETY TIP
Don't lock your elbows

Tricep dips
Areas trained: Rear upper arms, shoulders

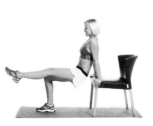

» Begin seated on a chair, placing your hands just outside your thighs. Walk your feet forward, coming off the chair so your body weight is supported by your hands and feet.
» Lift your left foot off the floor and straighten your knee.
» Lower yourself towards the floor so your elbows are bent at 90 degrees, push through your hands to straighten your arms and repeat.
» Continue for the allotted time, changing feet halfway through.

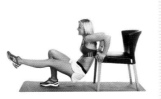

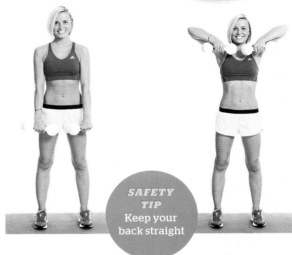

SAFETY TIP
Keep your back straight

Upright row
Areas trained:
Shoulders, upper back

» Begin standing with feet hip-width apart, holding a 4-8kg dumbbell in each hand with your hands by your thighs.
» Bring your hands up towards your shoulders, taking your elbows upwards and outwards.
» Slowly straighten your arms and return to the start. Repeat.

🕐 **11am** 1-hour hot yoga class

🕐 **2pm** Lower-body toning session

Beginner	Intermediate	Advanced
Choose 4 exercises and complete 2 circuits, **perform each exercise for 30 secs**	Choose 5 exercises and complete 2 circuits, **perform each exercise for 45 secs**	Complete 2 circuits of all exercises, **perform each exercise for 1 min**

Walking lunges
Areas trained: Thighs, bottom

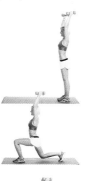

» Stand with feet hip-width apart holding a light dumbbell in each hand above your head with hands slightly wider than shoulder-width apart.
» Take a large step forward with your left foot then lunge down, bending both knees and lowering down until your back knee is just above the floor.
» Straighten your legs and take a large step forward with your right foot and repeat. Continue alternating legs.

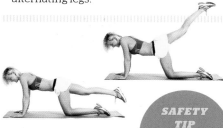

Donkey kicks
Areas trained:
Bottom, rear thighs

SAFETY TIP
Keep your back straight

» Begin on all fours then extend your right leg out behind you, slightly off the floor.
» Raise your leg, keeping it straight so your foot is just higher than your hips, squeezing your bottom as you do so.
» Lower to just above the ground and repeat.
» Change legs halfway through each set.

SAFETY TIP
Don't allow your back to arch

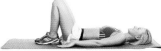
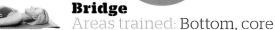

Bridge
Areas trained: Bottom, core

» Lie on your back with knees bent, feet flat on the floor and arms by your sides.
» Tighten your stomach and lift your hips off the floor into a bridge position with your body in a straight line from your shoulders to knees.
» Straighten your left leg, keeping your hips level. Hold, then lower your body back down to the floor and repeat.
» Change legs halfway through each set.

Stability ball leg curl
Areas trained: Rear thighs, bottom, lower back

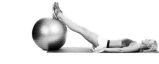
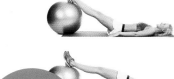
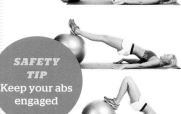

SAFETY TIP
Keep your abs engaged

» Begin lying on your back, feet resting on a stability ball, arms by your sides.
» Lift your hips to form a straight line from your ankles to your shoulders.
» Maintaining this position, bend your knees to roll the ball towards you.
» Slowly straighten your knees and lower your hips to the floor. Repeat.

Jump squat
Areas trained: Front thighs, bottom

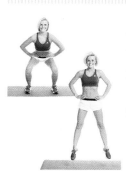

» Stand with your feet shoulder-width apart, hands on your hips.
» Bend your hips and knees and squat down as if you were going to sit on a chair behind you, without leaning excessively forward from the hips.
» Quickly straighten your legs, jumping as high as you can, landing softly then returning to the start position. Repeat.

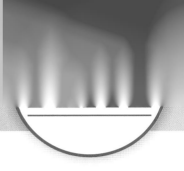

Squat thrusts
Areas trained: Thighs, bottom, shoulders, core

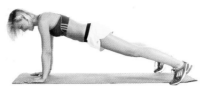

» Start in plank position with shoulders over hands, tummy tight and body in a straight line from shoulders to feet.
» Jump your feet out to the sides and back together, then jump your feet forward towards your hands, bending your knees to a crouching position.
» Jump your feet back to the start and repeat.

SAFETY TIP
Keep your back straight

SAFETY TIP
Keep the knee of the straight leg soft, not locked

Leg raises
Area trained: Bottom

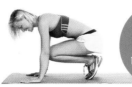

» Lie on your side with your upper body supported by your elbow, lower leg bent and upper leg straight.
» Lift your upper leg slightly off the floor – this is your starting position.
» Raise your upper leg to around 45 degrees, then slowly lower back to the start and repeat.
» Turn onto the other side and repeat with the other leg halfway through each set.

Wall sit
Area trained: Front thighs

» Place a stability ball against a wall and rest against it, facing away from the wall so your lower back is supported and your hips and knees are bent to 90 degrees.
» Hold this position for the allotted time.

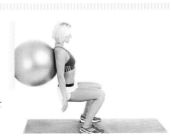

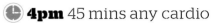

⏱ **4pm** 45 mins any cardio

⏱ **5pm** Core and tummy toning session (complete the following circuit)

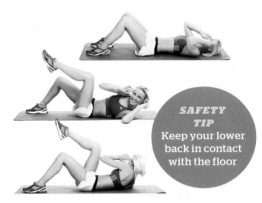

SAFETY TIP
Keep your lower back in contact with the floor

Twisting crunch
Area trained: Stomach

» Lie on your back with your feet flat on the floor, hips and knees bent, hands lightly touching your temples.
» Slowly lift your shoulders off the floor and twist your upper body to the left, taking your right shoulder towards your left knee, while simultaneously drawing your left knee in towards your elbow.
» Lower yourself back down and repeat, twisting to the right.

Beginner	Intermediate	Advanced
2 sets of 10 reps	2 sets of 16 reps	3 sets of 16-20 reps
5 twists each side	**8 twists each side**	**8-10 twists each side**

Reverse crunch
Area trained: Lower stomach

» Lie on your back with your feet off the floor, hips and knees bent at 90 degrees, thighs pressed together, and arms by your sides.
» Raise your hips off the floor towards your ribs, concentrating on using your lower stomach to create the movement.
» Lower your body back to the starting position, allowing your hips to lightly touch the floor, then repeat.

SAFETY TIP
Keep your neck relaxed throughout and perform the move with control

Beginner	Intermediate	Advanced
2 sets of **8-12 reps**	3 sets of **10-12 reps**	3 sets of **12-15 reps**

Russian twist
Areas trained: Upper stomach, sides of stomach

» Sit on the floor with your hips and knees bent and your arms straight out in front of you. Lean back to 45 degrees.
» Twist to the left and pause, return to the centre and twist to the right to complete one rep. Repeat for half of the prescribed reps.
» Lower your torso slightly further, twisting to the right, and then left to complete one set.

Beginner	Intermediate	Advanced
2 sets of **6-8 reps**	2 sets of **8-10 reps**	2 sets of **10-12 reps**

SAFETY TIP
Keep your back straight

Beginner	Intermediate	Advanced
2 sets of **10 reps 1-sec hold**	2 sets of **10 reps 2-sec hold**	2 sets of **10 reps 3-sec hold**

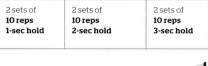
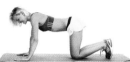
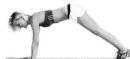

Knee lift
Areas trained: Core, stomach, shoulders

» Begin on all fours. Exhale, tightening your abs and engaging your pelvic floor muscles, lifting your knees off the floor and holding for the allotted time for your level.
» Lower slowly to the floor and repeat.

SAFETY TIP
Don't allow your back to arch

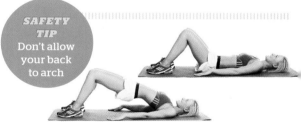

Beginner	Intermediate	Advanced
2 sets of **8-10 reps**	2 sets of **10-12 reps**	2 sets of **12-15 reps**

Hip bridge
Areas trained: Core, stomach, bottom

» Lie flat on your back with knees bent and feet flat on the floor, arms by your sides.
» Tighten your stomach and engage your pelvic floor muscles, lifting your hips to form a straight line from your shoulders to your knees.
» Hold for a count of two, lower and repeat.

48-hour fat attack diet plan

🕐 **7am** Lemon cleanse
» 1 glass of room-temperature water
with a squeeze of lemon

🕐 **7.30am** Breakfast
» Breakfast boost juice (p121)
» Supplements

🕐 **11am** Snack
» 1 apple and 2 tablespoons of mixed raw
nuts and/or seeds

🕐 **2pm** Lunch
» Carrot soup (p123)

🕐 **5pm** Snack
» 2 tablespoons of mixed raw nuts and/or seeds
and 2 handfuls of blueberries

🕐 **7pm** Dinner
» Lovely lettuce soup (p122)

🕐 **10pm** Overnight detox drink
» 1 cup of instant miso soup

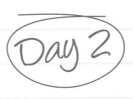

Day 2

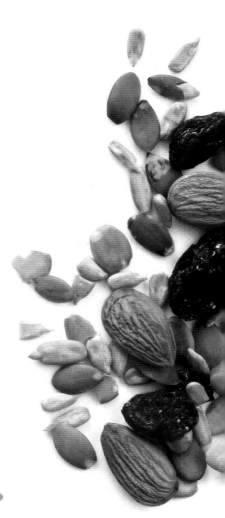

48-hour fat attack workout plan

🕐 9am 30-minute interval run

Beginner	Intermediate	Advanced
1-min walk	2-min jog	1-min jog
1-min jog	1-min sprint	1-min run
x15	**x10**	1-min sprint
		x10

🕐 10am 1-hour Pilates class or DVD

🕐 1pm Circuit training

Beginner	Intermediate	Advanced
4 circuits **30 secs each exercise**	5 circuits **45 secs each exercise**	5 circuits **1 min each exercise**

Treadmills
Areas trained:
Cardio, thighs

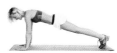
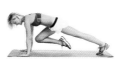
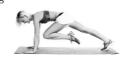

» Begin in plank position, holding your core tight.
» Step your right foot forward towards your right hand.
» Quickly reverse feet, jumping your right foot back and left foot forward. Continue alternating feet as quickly as you can.

Push-up burpees
Areas trained: Cardio, thighs, bottom, chest, shoulders, rear upper arms, stomach

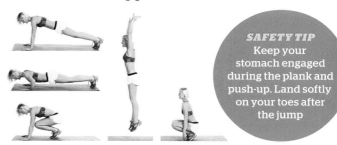

SAFETY TIP
Keep your stomach engaged during the plank and push-up. Land softly on your toes after the jump

» Begin in plank position, shoulders over hands, tummy tight and your body in a straight line.
» Then lower your chest to the floor, performing a push-up. Straighten your arms and return to plank position.
» Jump your feet towards your hands, then jump straight up, taking your arms up over your head.
» Land softly and squat down, placing your hands either side of your feet, then jump your feet back into plank position. This is one rep. Repeat for duration.

Star jump burpee
Area trained: Cardio

» From plank position, jump your feet towards your hands, then jump up, performing a star jump.
» Land softly with your feet together, then jump back into plank position and repeat the move (see move above).

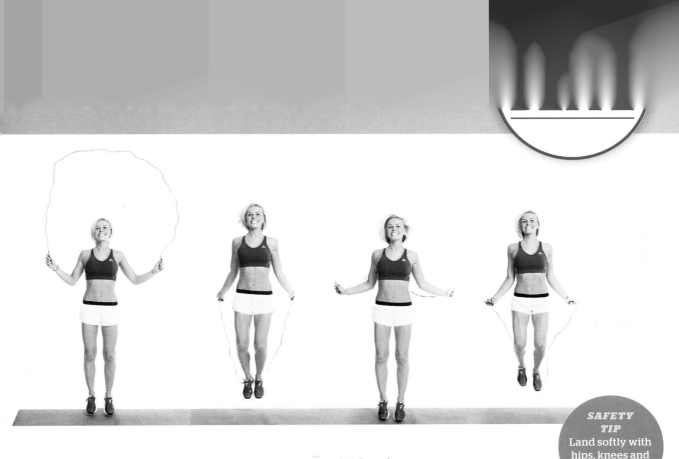

SAFETY TIP
Land softly with hips, knees and ankles aligned

Jump squat
Areas trained: Front thighs, bottom, calves

» Stand with your feet shoulder-width apart, hands on your hips.

» Simultaneously bend your hips and knees and squat down as if you were going to sit on a chair behind you, without leaning forward excessively from the hips.

» Quickly straighten your legs, jumping as high as you can, landing softly then returning to standing. Repeat.

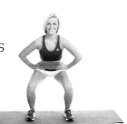

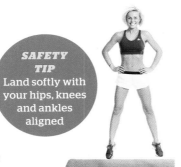

SAFETY TIP
Land softly with your hips, knees and ankles aligned

Skipping
Areas trained: Thighs, calves, shoulders, cardio

» Remember to only jump high enough to allow the rope to pass under your feet, performing as many revolutions of the rope as you can in the allotted time. Adjust the length of the rope so that when standing on the centre, the handles just reach your underarms.

4pm 1-hour any cardio or class

Congratulations, you're done! Hopefully, you're feeling great and your belly is looking flat! »

Your results

Track your progress on the 48-hour fat attack plan

	Before	After
Weight		
Arms		
Bust		
Waist		
Hips		
Thighs		

Great result! Why not try the 7-day slim-down?

1-week
waist away plan

Perfect for a quick-fix bikini body

Get ready to show off your tummy after you blitz through this fast and effective programme

Be sure to fill in your vital statistics on page 65, so you can measure your results

Caution: As with any diet, you should consult your doctor before starting this plan and if you experience any unpleasant symptoms you should stop the diet and see a healthcare professional immediately. This plan is not suitable for those who are underweight, pregnant or planning on becoming pregnant, or breastfeeding. This plan should not be followed for more than one week.

Things to remember

You'll lose inches on this week-long plan if you follow the rules closely!

Equipment you'll need
» Juicer to juice fruits and vegetables
» Blender or hand blender for soups

» This slim-down plan is designed to target your mid-section – that bit you'll be showing off in a bikini! It may not seem like a huge amount of time but you'll be surprised at what you can achieve in a week if you make exercising and eating right your main priorities. In seven days you could lose between one and three inches from your waist! This diet is low-carb, not no-carb. It includes lots of fruit and veg plus lean protein to keep your metabolism revving.

The rules

» Days 1 and 2 are detox days. On these days, breakfast is a juice; lunch and dinner are soups. The morning and afternoon snacks are 2 tablespoons of nuts and seeds, and fruit. The day ends with a detox drink, which is a light miso soup.

» From day 3 you replace the lunchtime soup with a salad and the dinner soup with lean protein and veggies. When the plan says salad you can have unlimited amounts of salad leaves and non-root veggies, although you must limit the dressing to two tablespoons. The morning snack is a piece of fruit plus nuts and seeds, and the afternoon snack is yoghurt and fruit. You drop the miso soup on day 3. From day 3 onwards if you need post-workout replenishment, have a protein bar or protein shake.

» Drink 1.5 litres of water each day.

» Take the following supplements every morning with your breakfast:
» Multivitamin/mineral
» Omega-3
» Mixed antioxidants

» Exercise and relax. Follow the exercise plan for each day. Aim to sleep at least seven hours a night. You may also want to have a nap during the day.

» Don't drink coffee, tea, cola or other caffeinated drinks, including green tea. Replace them with water, or herbal teas and decaf coffee without milk.

» Don't drink alcohol of any kind. Don't drink fruit juice, smoothies or fruit cordials. The only juices you should drink are those you have made according to the recipes on the plan.

» Don't eat any starchy carbs such as bread, pasta, rice, potatoes, cakes and biscuits.

» No chocolate!

1-week **waist away diet plan**

🕐 **7am** Lemon cleanse
» 1 glass of room-temperature water with a squeeze of lemon

🕐 **7.30am** Breakfast
» 1 beetroot liver cleanse juice (p120)
» Supplements

🕐 **10.30am** Snack
» 1 apple and 2 tablespoons of mixed raw nuts and/or seeds (Brazil nuts, almonds, walnuts and pumpkin or sunflower seeds)

🕐 **1pm** Lunch
» Green goddess soup (p122)

🕐 **4pm** Snack
» 2 tablespoons of mixed raw nuts and/or seeds and 2 handfuls of blueberries

🕐 **7pm** Dinner
» Cauliflower detox soup (p122)

🕐 **10pm** Overnight detox drink
» 1 cup of instant miso soup

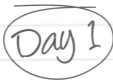

Day 1

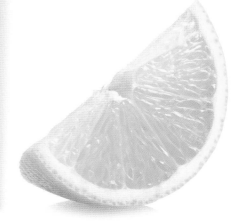

1-week waist away workout plan

⏱ **8.30am** Complete the following circuit:

Beginner	Intermediate	Advanced
30 secs each exercise, **repeat 4 times**	45 secs each exercise, **repeat 4 times**	60 secs each exercise, **repeat 4 times**

Plank
Areas trained: Abs, lower back

» Begin on all fours then tighten your stomach and walk your feet back into plank position. Your body should form a straight line from shoulders to feet.
» Hold this position for the allotted time for your level.

Jumping lunges
Areas trained: Thighs, bottom

» Begin standing with one foot in front of the other, then bend your knees and lower into a lunge.
» Quickly jump up and switch legs in the air, then lunge down. Repeat for the allotted time.

Scissors
Area trained: Lower stomach

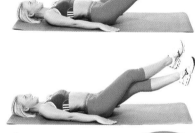

» Lie on your back with your arms on the floor by your sides, legs outstretched at a height you can hold without arching your back.
» Take your left leg over your right so they cross, then apart, and then bring your right leg over your left.
» Continue for the allotted time.

SAFETY TIP
Make sure your front knee stays behind your toes and directly above your ankle

SAFETY TIP
Keep your lower back in contact with the floor

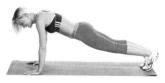

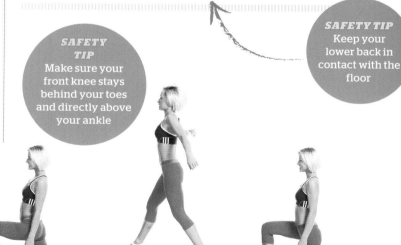

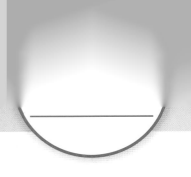

Side jumps
Areas trained: Thighs, calves

» Stand to one side of an imaginary line. Jump with both feet to the other side, then immediately back again. Continue jumping for the allotted time.

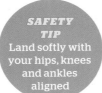

SAFETY TIP
Land softly with your hips, knees and ankles aligned

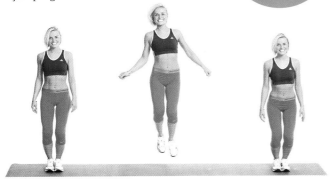

Push-up burpees
Areas trained: Cardio, thighs, bottom, chest, shoulders, rear upper arms, stomach

» Begin in plank position, then lower your chest to the floor, performing a push-up. Straighten your arms and return to plank position.
» Jump your feet towards your hands, then jump straight up, taking your arms up over your head.
» Land softly and squat down, placing your hands either side of your feet, then jump your feet back into plank. This is one rep. Repeat for the allotted time.

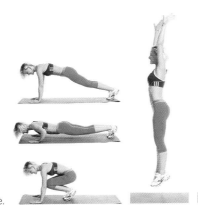

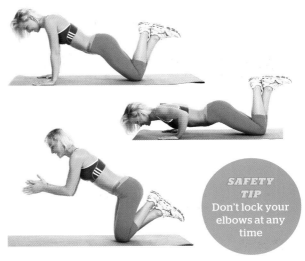

SAFETY TIP
Don't lock your elbows at any time

Explosive push-up
Areas trained: Chest, shoulders, rear upper arms

» Begin in a box or modified push-up position, hands slightly wider than shoulder-width apart.
» Lower your chest to just above the floor.
» As quickly and powerfully as you can, push through your hands, straightening your arms and taking your hands off the floor momentarily.
» Place your hands back on the floor and repeat the move for the allotted time.
» To increase the challenge, clap your hands together when they leave the floor.

Plus
» Running or swimming

Beginner	Intermediate	Advanced
30 mins	40 mins	50 mins

1-week **waist away diet plan**

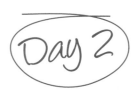 *Day 2*

🕐 **7am** Lemon cleanse
» 1 glass of room-temperature water with a squeeze of lemon

🕐 **7.30am** Breakfast
» 1 breakfast boost juice (p121)
» Supplements

🕐 **10.30am** Snack
» 1 apple and 2 tablespoons of mixed raw nuts and/or seeds

🕐 **1pm** Lunch
» Carrot soup (p123)

🕐 **4pm** Snack
» 2 tablespoons of mixed raw nuts and/or seeds and 2 handfuls of blueberries

🕐 **7pm** Dinner
» Lovely lettuce soup (p122)

🕐 **10pm** Overnight detox drink
» 1 cup instant miso soup

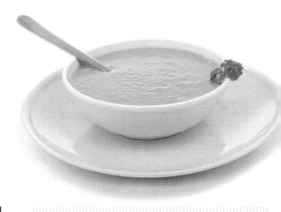

1-week **waist away workout plan**

🕐 **9am** Any cardio

Beginner	Intermediate	Advanced
30 mins	45 mins	60 mins
7/10 intensity	**8/10 intensity**	**8/10 intensity**

🕐 **7.30am** Breakfast
» 1 vitamin vitality juice (p120)
» Supplements

🕐 **10.30am** Snack
» 1 apple and 1 tablespoon of mixed raw nuts and/or seeds

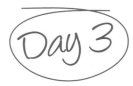 *Day 3*

🕐 **1pm** Lunch
» Tandoori chicken salad (p124)

🕐 **4pm** Snack
» 1 small fat-free Greek yoghurt with half a pack of berries

🕐 **7pm** Dinner
» Stuffed mushrooms (p128)

1-week waist away workout plan

9am Complete the following circuit:

Push-up

Areas trained: Shoulders, chest, rear upper arms

» Begin in a box or modified push-up position, hands slightly wider than shoulder-width apart.
» Keeping your tummy tight, lower your chest to just above the floor.
» Straighten your arms and return to the start, then repeat.

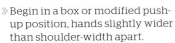
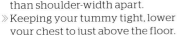

SAFETY TIP
Don't lock your elbows

Beginner	Intermediate	Advanced
2 sets of **10 reps**	2 sets of **12 reps**	2 sets of **15 reps**

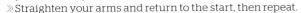

Diamond press-up

Areas trained: Shoulders chest, rear upper arms

» Begin in a full or modified push-up position with hands under your chest. Your left and right index fingers and thumbs should touch to form a diamond shape.
» Keeping your body in a straight line, bend your arms and lower your chest to an inch off the floor.
» Pause for one second then straighten your arms and return to the start.

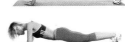

Beginner	Intermediate	Advanced
2 sets of **10 reps**	2 sets of **12 reps**	2 sets of **15 reps**

SAFETY TIP
Don't lock your elbows or allow your hips to sag

Jump squat

Areas trained: Front thighs, bottom

» Stand with feet shoulder-width apart, hands on hips.
» Simultaneously bend your hips and knees and squat down as if you were going to sit on a chair behind you, without leaning forward excessively from the hips.
» Quickly straighten your legs, jumping as high as you can, landing softly then return to standing. Repeat.
» To increase the difficulty hold a dumbbell or weight in each hand, with your arms by your sides throughout.

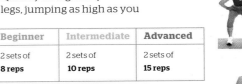
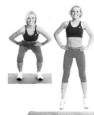

Beginner	Intermediate	Advanced
2 sets of **8 reps**	2 sets of **10 reps**	2 sets of **15 reps**

Crunch

Area trained: Stomach

» Begin lying on your back with your legs pointing straight up towards the ceiling and your arms across your chest
» Crunch up, taking your shoulders towards your thighs.
» Return to the start and repeat.

Beginner	Intermediate	Advanced
3 sets of **8-10 reps**	3 sets of **10-12 reps**	3 sets of **15-20 reps**

Push-up burpees

Areas trained: Cardio, thighs, bottom, chest, shoulders, rear upper arms, stomach

» Begin in plank position, shoulders over hands and your body in a straight line.
» Lower your chest to the floor, performing a push-up. Straighten your arms and return to plank position.
» Jump your feet towards your hands, then jump up, taking your arms upward.
» Land softly and squat down, placing your hands either side of your feet, then jump your feet back into plank. This is one rep. Repeat to complete set.

Beginner	Intermediate	Advanced
2 sets of **12 reps**	2 sets of **15 reps**	2 sets of **20 reps**

> **SAFETY TIP**
> Ensure your knees are aligned over your toes. Keep your back straight and abs tight

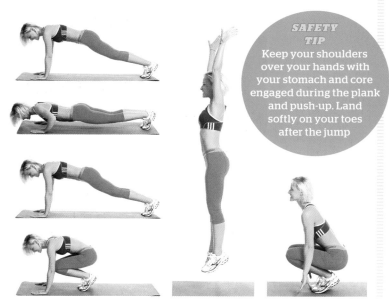

> **SAFETY TIP**
> Keep your shoulders over your hands with your stomach and core engaged during the plank and push-up. Land softly on your toes after the jump

Plié squat

Areas trained: Inner thighs, bottom

» Stand with feet slightly wider than hip-width apart, toes turned out, hands on hips.
» Keeping your tummy tight, squat deeply so that your hips are level with your knees.
» Push through your heels and return to standing, without locking your knees, then repeat.

Beginner	Intermediate	Advanced
2 sets of **10 reps**	2 sets of **12 reps**	2 sets of **15 reps**

Plus
High-intensity intervals

Any cardio: 10/10 intensity for 20 secs, then 6/10 intensity for 10 secs

Beginner	Intermediate	Advanced
Repeat x 8	Repeat x 10	Repeat x 12

1-week waist away diet plan

🕐 **7.30am** Breakfast
» 1 sunrise juice (p120)
» Supplements

🕐 **10.30am** Snack
» 1 apple and 1 tablespoon of mixed raw nuts and/or seeds

🕐 **1pm** Lunch
» Feta and mint salad (p124)

🕐 **4pm** Snack
» 1 small fat-free Greek yoghurt with half a pack of berries

🕐 **7pm** Dinner Cauliflower pizza (p126)

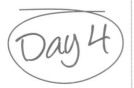

Day 4

1-week waist away workout plan

🕐 **6pm** Any cardio

Beginner	Intermediate	Advanced
40 mins	60 mins	75 mins
7/10 intensity	**8/10 intensity**	**8/10 intensity**

1-week waist away diet plan

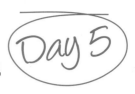

Day 5

🕐 **7.30am** Breakfast
» 1 green pineapple juice (p120)
» Supplements

🕐 **10.30am** Snack
» 1 apple and 1 tablespoon of mixed raw nuts and/or seeds

🕐 **1pm** Lunch
» Tuna Niçoise salad (p124)

🕐 **4pm** Snack
» 1 small fat-free Greek yoghurt with half a pack of berries

🕐 **7pm** Dinner
» California omelette (p126)

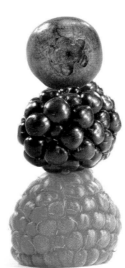

1-week waist away workout plan

🕐 **6pm** Repeat day 1 circuit (p58)
Plus
High-intensity intervals
Any cardio: 10/10 intensity for 20 secs, then 6/10 intensity for 10 secs

Beginner	Intermediate	Advanced
Repeat x 8	Repeat x 10	Repeat x 12

1-week waist away diet plan

Day 6

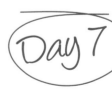

🕑 **7.30am** Breakfast
» 1 tomato and celery juice (p120)
» Supplements

🕑 **10.30am** Snack
» 1 apple and 1 tablespoon mixed raw nuts and/or seeds

🕑 **1pm** Lunch
» Tandoori chicken salad (p124)

🕑 **4pm** Snack
» 1 small fat-free Greek yoghurt with half a pack of berries

🕑 **7pm** Dinner
» Stuffed mushrooms (p128)

1-week waist away workout plan

🕑 **6pm** Any cardio

Beginner	Intermediate	Advanced
40 mins **7/10 intensity**	60 mins **8/10 intensity**	75 mins **8/10 intensity**

1-week waist away diet plan

🕑 **7.30am** Breakfast
» 1 morning refresher juice (p120)
» Supplements

🕑 **10.30am** Snack
» 1 apple and 1 tablespoon of mixed raw nuts and/or seeds

🕑 **1pm** Lunch
» Cottage cheese salad (p128)

🕑 **4pm** Snack
» 1 small fat-free Greek yoghurt with half a pack of berries

🕑 **7pm** Dinner
» Cod with stir-fried vegetables (p130)

Day 7

1-week waist away workout plan

🕑 **9am** Repeat day 3 circuit (p61)

Your results

Track your progress on the 1-week waist away plan

	Before	After
Weight		
Arms		
Bust		
Waist		
Hips		
Thighs		

It was a tough week, but you made it! Hopefully you're now feeling svelte and sexy

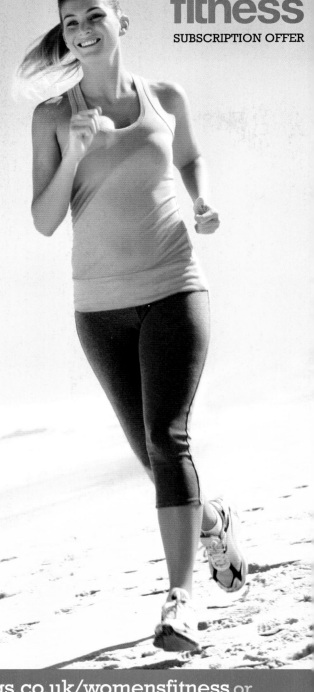

women's fitness
SUBSCRIPTION OFFER

Special offer!

Try 3 issues for just £1

3 ISSUES FOR £1

If you want to learn how to fit regular excerise into your hectic routine without resorting to crash diets, extreme exercise plans or long, exhausting workouts, then *Women's Fitness* is the magazine for you.

SUBSCRIBE TODAY & RECEIVE:

- ☑ Your first **3 issues for £1**
- ☑ **30% saving** on all subsequent issues
- ☑ **FREE delivery** direct to your door
- ☑ **Inspiring and motivating features** to get you moving and staying active.

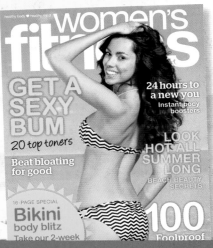

Order online at **www.dennismags.co.uk/womensfitness** or

CALL 0844 844 0246

using offer code: **G1207HBC**

14-day

drop a dress size plan

Try the fortnight fix

Get serious results in a seriously short time with this clever plan

Be sure to fill in your vital statistics on page 90, so you can measure your results

Caution: As with any diet, you should consult your doctor before starting this plan and if you experience any unpleasant symptoms you should stop the diet and see a healthcare professional immediately. This plan is not suitable for those who are underweight, pregnant or planning on becoming pregnant, or breastfeeding. This plan should not be followed for more than two weeks.

Things to remember

Two weeks is plenty of time to make a serious difference. Follow these rules for real success

>> If you've got a bit more time to play with, try this 14-day bootcamp. It still incorporates a detox element to reduce bloating and flush out water, however, you also have the opportunity to shift some significant fat. Over the course of two weeks, you could drop as much as a dress size if you stick to the plan and really get going on the exercise.

The plan zigzags between low-calorie and high-calorie days to constantly shock your body into burning fat. It begins with a two-day detox, then five days when you can add in some lean protein and dairy. Then it's back to a two-day detox, before you go back to lean protein, dairy and some beans. The beans are important because they help hormone balance, which is key to reducing fat storage, especially around the stomach, and they'll give you energy to work out hard. In addition to the workouts, try to be as active as you can every day. Taking the stairs wherever you can may only take a few extra seconds, but every calorie counts!

Equipment you'll need
» Juicer to juice fruits and vegetables
» Blender or hand blender for soups
» 2 x 4-8kg dumbbells
» 2 x 3-5kg dumbbells
» 5-8kg medicine ball
» Resistance band
» Stability ball
» 2 water bottles
» Skipping rope
» Step

The rules

» Days 1 and 2 of both weeks are detox days. On these days, breakfast is a juice, and lunch and dinner are soups. The morning and afternoon snacks are two tablespoons of nuts and seeds plus fruit. The day ends with an overnight detox drink, which is a light miso soup.

» For days 3 to 7, the lunchtime soup is replaced with a salad and the dinner soup with a cooked meal. When the plan says salad you can have unlimited amounts of salad leaves and non-root veggies, although you must limit the dressing to two tablespoons. The morning snack is a piece of fruit and nuts and seeds and the afternoon snack is yoghurt and fruit.

» For days 10 to 14, lean protein, dairy and a small portion of beans are reintroduced to your diet. Breakfast is a homemade juice; the morning snack is a piece of fruit with nuts and seeds; lunch is a salad; the afternoon snack is fat-free Greek yoghurt with fresh berries and the evening meal contains protein and beans. On non-detox days if you need post-workout replenishment to aid your recovery, have a protein bar or shake.

» Drink 1.5 litres of water each day.

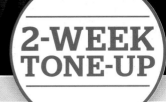

14-day drop a dress size diet plan

» Take the following supplements every morning with your breakfast:
» Multivitamin/mineral
» Omega-3
» Mixed antioxidants

» Exercise and relax. Follow the exercise plan for each day. Aim to sleep at least seven hours a night. You may also want to have a nap during detox days.

» Don't drink coffee, tea, cola or other caffeinated drinks, including green tea. Replace them with water, or herbal teas and decaf coffee without milk.

» Don't drink alcohol of any kind. Don't drink fruit juice, smoothies or fruit cordials. The only juices you should drink are those you have made according to the recipes on the plan.

» Don't eat any starchy carbs such as bread, pasta, rice, potatoes, cakes and biscuits.

» No chocolate!

7am Lemon cleanse
» 1 glass of room-temperature water with a squeeze of lemon

7.30am Breakfast
» 1 beetroot liver cleanse juice (p120)
» Supplements

10.30am Snack
» 1 apple and 2 tablespoons of mixed raw nuts and/or seeds (Brazil nuts, almonds and pumpkin seeds)

1pm Lunch
» Green goddess soup (p122)

4pm Snack
» 2 tablespoons of mixed raw nuts and/or seeds and 2 handfuls of blueberries

7pm Dinner
» Cauliflower detox soup (p122)

10pm Overnight detox drink
» 1 cup of instant miso soup

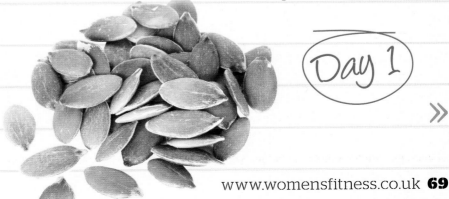

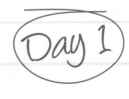

Day 1

14-day drop a dress size workout plan

🕐 2pm Interval training

Beginner	Intermediate	Advanced
1-min walk	2-min jog	1-min jog
1-min jog	1-min sprint	2-min run
x15	**x10**	**x10**

🕐 6pm Plyometric circuit

Find your level

Beginner: Complete the following circuit 8 times, performing each exercise for 30 secs

Intermediate: Complete the circuit 10 times, performing each exercise for 45 secs

Advanced: Complete the circuit 10 times, performing each exercise for 1 min

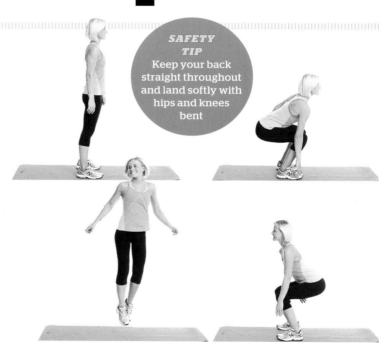

SAFETY TIP
Keep your back straight throughout and land softly with hips and knees bent

Snowboarder
Areas trained: Cardio, thighs, bottom

» Begin with your right foot in front of your left, body turned to the left and feet angled at around 45 degrees, as if you were on a snowboard.
» Slowly squat down, bringing your right hand to the floor.

» Jump up, alternating your feet and landing so your left foot is in front of your right with body turned to the right.
» Continue for the allotted time for your level, alternating direction with each rep.

Mountain climbers
Areas trained: Cardio, thighs

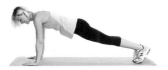
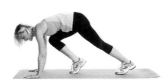
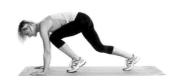

» From plank position, walk your feet towards your hands so your hips are higher than your shoulders, then bring your right foot forward towards your hands – this is your starting position.
» Jump with both feet, bringing them off the floor and land with feet alternated, then repeat immediately.
» Continue for the allotted time.

Skipping jacks
Areas trained: Cardio, thighs, calves

» While skipping, alternate landing with feet together and feet wider than shoulder-width apart with each skip for the allotted time.

SAFETY TIP
Land softly on the balls of your feet

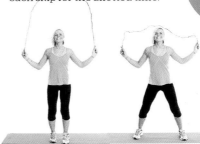

High knees
Areas trained: Cardio, thighs

» Begin jogging on the spot then bring your knees up level with your hips with each step, driving your arms back and forth in a running motion.

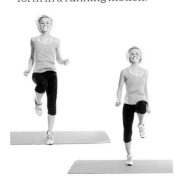

Striding jumps
Areas trained: Cardio, thighs, bottom

» Begin with your left foot on a step or bench, then push through your right foot, jumping up and alternating legs so your right foot is on the step.
» Continue, alternating legs, jumping as soon as your foot makes contact with the step.

SAFETY TIP
Land softly with knees in line with ankles

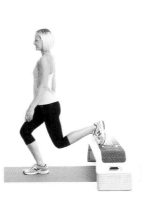
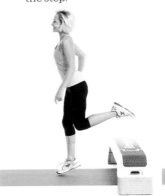
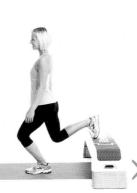

14-day drop a dress size diet plan

🕐 **7am** Lemon cleanse
» 1 glass of room-temperature water with a squeeze of lemon

🕐 **7.30am** Breakfast
» 1 breakfast boost juice (p121)
» Supplements

🕐 **10.30am** Snack
» 1 apple and 2 tablespoons of mixed raw nuts and/or seeds

🕐 **1pm** Lunch
» Carrot soup (p123)

🕐 **4pm** Snack
» 2 tablespoons of mixed raw nuts and/or seeds and 2 handfuls of blueberries

🕐 **7pm** Dinner
» Lovely lettuce soup (p122)

🕐 **10pm** Overnight detox drink
» 1 cup of instant miso soup

14-day drop a dress size workout plan

🕐 **Rest day**, all levels

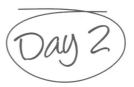

14-day drop a dress size workout plan

🕐 **2pm** 1-hour yoga class, all levels

🕐 **6pm** 1-hour any cardio or class, all levels

🕐 **7.30am** Breakfast
» 1 vitamin vitality juice (p120)
» Supplements

🕐 **10.30am** Snack
» 1 apple and 1 tablespoon of mixed raw nuts and/or seeds

🕐 **1pm** Lunch
» Tandoori chicken salad (p124)

🕐 **4pm** Snack
» 1 small fat-free Greek yoghurt with half a pack of berries

🕐 **7pm** Dinner
» Stuffed mushrooms (p128)

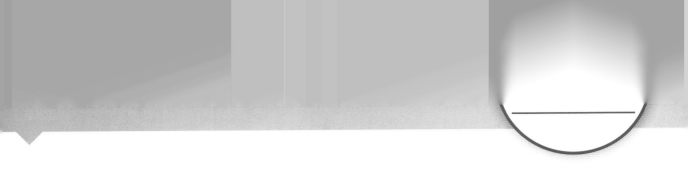

14-day drop a dress size diet plan

🕐 **7.30am** Breakfast
» 1 sunrise juice (p120)
» Supplements

🕐 **10.30am** Snack
» 1 apple and 1 tablespoon of mixed raw nuts and/or seeds

🕐 **1pm** Lunch
» Feta and mint salad (p124)

🕐 **4pm** Snack
» 1 small fat-free Greek yoghurt with half a pack of berries

🕐 **7pm** Dinner
» Cauliflower pizza (p126)

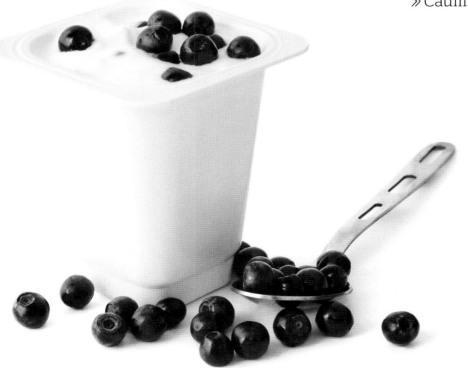

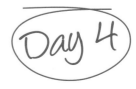

Day 4

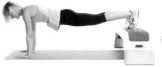
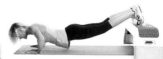

14-day drop a dress size workout plan

🕑 **2pm** Interval training

Beginner	Intermediate	Advanced
1-min walk	2-min jog	1-min jog
1-min jog	1-min sprint	2-min run
x15	**x10**	**x10**

🕑 **6pm** Upper-body toning circuit

Find your level

Beginner: Choose 5 exercises and complete 2 circuits, performing each exercise for 30 secs

Intermediate: Choose 7 exercises and complete 2 circuits, performing each exercise for 45 secs

Advanced: Complete 2 circuits of all exercises, performing each exercise for 1 min

Incline push-up
Areas trained: Upper chest, shoulders, rear upper arms

» Begin in a full or modified push-up position with your hands just wider than shoulder-width apart and your feet on a step or box.
» Bend your elbows and lower your chest to an inch above the ground, keeping your body in a straight line from shoulders to feet.
» Push through your hands, straightening your arms and returning to the start position. Repeat.

> **SAFETY TIP**
> Keep your abs tight and don't let your hips sag

Medicine ball pull-over
Areas trained: Chest, shoulders, upper back

» Sit on a stability ball holding a 5-8kg medicine ball with hands shoulder-width apart, and walk your feet forward until only your head, neck and upper back are supported, with your knees bent at 90 degrees.
» Keeping your stomach tight, lift the medicine ball until it's directly over your chest, keeping your arms extended straight – this is your starting position.
» Slowly extend your arms straight behind you, in line with your body, with upper arms close to your ears.
» Slowly raise your arms to the starting position and repeat for duration.

> **SAFETY TIP**
> Keep your back straight throughout

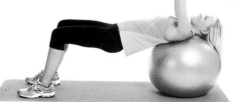
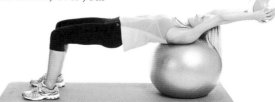

Plank transfer
Areas trained: Shoulders, core, rear upper arms

» Begin in plank position, resting on your forearms, your stomach tight and body in a straight line from feet to shoulders.

» Transfer your weight slightly to your right side, straightening your left arm, placing your hand on the floor under your shoulder. Repeat with your right arm to come into a full push-up position.

» Hold for a count of one then return to resting on your forearms, one arm at a time, to complete one rep. Repeat, starting with your right arm.

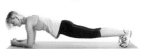
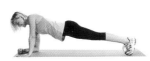
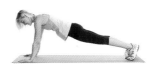

Bicep curl
Area trained: Front upper arms

» Stand with your feet shoulder-width apart, holding a 4-8kg dumbbell in each hand with your arms by your sides and palms facing forward.

» Bend your elbows, taking the dumbbells up towards your shoulders, keeping your elbows touching your sides with upper arms still.

» Lower the dumbbells down to the starting position and repeat the move.

Extra wide push-up
Areas trained: Chest, shoulders, rear upper arms

» Begin in a modified push-up position with your body in a straight line, hands under your shoulders and your arms around three inches wider than they would be for a regular push-up.

» Slowly and with control, lower your chest to just above the floor, then straighten your arms to return to the start. Repeat.

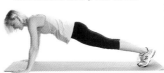
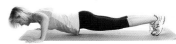

Tricep kickbacks
Area trained: Rear upper arms

» Stand with feet hip-width apart, holding a 3-5kg dumbbell in each hand by your sides.

» Bend forward 90 degrees from the hips, keeping your back straight and bending your elbows to 90 degrees so your forearms point towards the floor, your upper arms against your sides. This is your starting position.

» Slowly extend your elbows so your hands are level with your hips.

» Return to the start and repeat, keeping your upper arms still. Repeat.

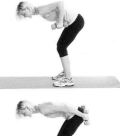
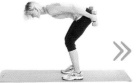

»

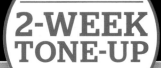

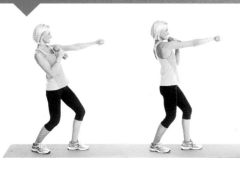

> **SAFETY TIP**
> Don't lock your elbows

Shadow boxing
Areas trained: Shoulders, arms

» Stand with your left foot slightly in front of your right and your left shoulder slightly in front of your right.
» Quickly punch straight ahead with your left hand, bringing it back and then repeating the punch with your right hand. Continue for the allotted time.
» Hold a dumbbell in each hand to increase the difficulty if required.

> **SAFETY TIP**
> Don't allow your elbows to bend to more than 90 degrees

Tricep dips
Areas trained: Rear upper arms, shoulders

» Begin seated on a chair, placing your hands just outside your thighs. Walk your feet forward, coming off the chair so your body weight is supported by your hands and feet.
» Lift your left foot off the floor and straighten your knee.
» Lower yourself towards the floor so your elbows are bent to 90 degrees, then push through your hands to straighten your arms and repeat the move.
» Continue for the allotted time, changing feet halfway through.

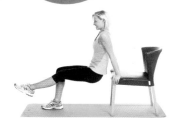

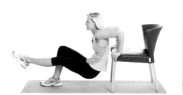

High row
Area trained: Upper back

» Begin seated with your legs straight out in front of you and a resistance band wrapped around your feet, holding an end in each hand. There should be a little tension in the band at this point.
» Bring your hands towards your shoulders, taking your elbows up and out so they are level with your shoulders. Return to the start and repeat.

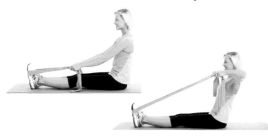

Upright row
Areas trained: Shoulders, upper back

» Begin standing with your feet hip-width apart, holding a 4-8kg dumbbell in each hand, by your thighs.
» Bring your hands up towards your shoulders, taking your elbows upwards and outwards.
» Slowly straighten your arms and return to the start. Repeat.

> **SAFETY TIP**
> Keep your back straight

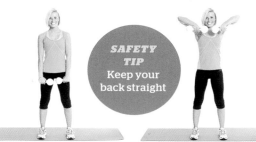

14-day **drop a dress size diet plan**

🕐 **7.30am** Breakfast
» 1 green pineapple juice (p120)
» Supplements

🕐 **10.30am** Snack
» 1 apple and 1 tablespoon of raw nuts and/or seeds

🕐 **1pm** Lunch
» Tuna Niçoise salad (p124)

🕐 **4pm** Snack
» 1 small fat-free Greek yoghurt with half a pack of berries

🕐 **7pm** Dinner
» California omelette (p126)

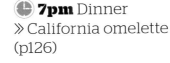

14-day **drop a dress size workout plan**

🕐 **5pm** 1-hour Pilates class or DVD, all levels

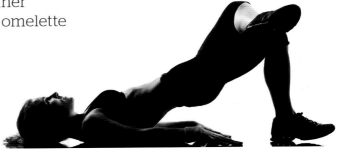

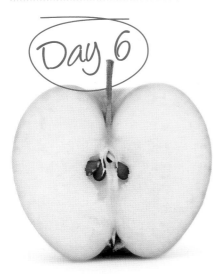

14-day **drop a dress size diet plan**

🕐 **7.30am** Breakfast
» 1 tomato and celery juice (p120)
» Supplements

🕐 **10.30am** Snack
» 1 apple and 1 tablespoon of raw nuts and/or seeds

🕐 **1pm** Lunch

» Cottage cheese salad (p128)

🕐 **4pm** Snack
» 1 fat-free Greek yoghurt with half a pack of berries

🕐 **7pm** Dinner
» Stuffed mushrooms (p128)

14-day drop a dress size workout plan

🕐 **8.30am** Interval training

Beginner	Intermediate	Advanced
1-min walk	2-min jog	1-min jog
1-min jog	1-min sprint	2-min run
x15	**x10**	**x10**

🕐 **9am** Lower-body toning circuit

Find your level

Beginner: Choose 4 exercises and complete 2 circuits, performing each exercise for 30 secs

Intermediate: Choose 5 exercises and complete 2 circuits, performing each exercise for 45 secs

Advanced: Complete 2 circuits of all exercises, performing each exercise for 1 min

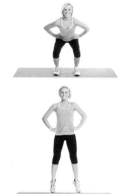

Jump squat
Areas trained:
Front thighs, bottom

» Stand with your feet shoulder-width apart, hands on your hips.
» Bend your hips and knees and squat down as if you were going to sit on a chair behind you, taking care not to lean too far forward from the hips.
» Quickly straighten your legs, jumping as high as you can, landing softly then returning to the start position. Repeat.

Walking lunges
Areas trained: Thighs, bottom

» Stand with feet hip-width apart holding a dumbbell in each hand above your head with arms straight and hands slightly wider than shoulder-width apart.
» Take a large step forward with your right foot then lunge down, bending both knees and lowering down until your back knee is just above the floor.
» Straighten your legs and take a large step forward with your left foot and repeat. Continue alternating legs.

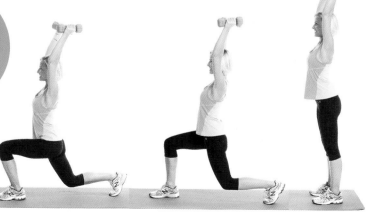

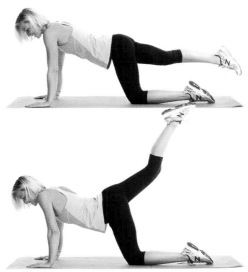

Donkey kicks
Areas trained:
Bottom, rear thighs

» Begin on all fours then extend your right leg out behind you, slightly off the floor.
» Raise your leg, keeping it straight so your foot is just higher than your hips, squeezing your bottom as you do so.
» Lower to just above the ground and repeat.
» Change legs halfway through each set.

SAFETY TIP
Keep your back straight

Squat thrusts
Areas trained:
Inner, outer and front thighs, bottom, shoulders, core

» Start in plank position with your shoulders over your hands, tummy tight and body in a straight line from shoulders to feet.
» Jump your feet out to the sides and back together, then jump your feet forward towards your hands, bending your knees.
» Jump your feet back to the start and repeat.

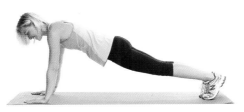

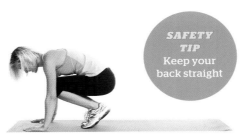

SAFETY TIP
Keep your back straight

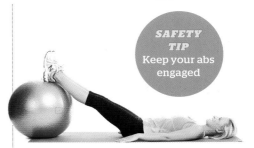

SAFETY TIP
Keep your abs engaged

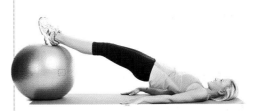

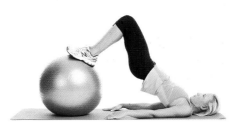

Stability ball leg curl
Areas trained: Rear thighs, bottom, lower back

» Begin lying on your back, feet resting on a stability ball, arms by your sides for support.
» Lift your hips to form a straight line between your knees and shoulders.
» Maintaining this position, bend your knees to roll the ball towards you.
» Slowly straighten your knees and lower your hips to the floor, and repeat.

Bridge
Areas trained: Bottom, core

» Lie on your back with knees bent and arms by your sides.
» Tighten your stomach and lift your hips off the floor into a bridge position with your body in a straight line.

» Straighten your left leg, keeping your hips level. Hold for a count of two, then lower your body back down and repeat.
» Change legs halfway through each set.

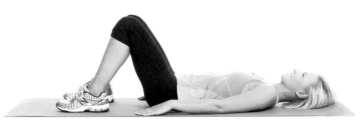

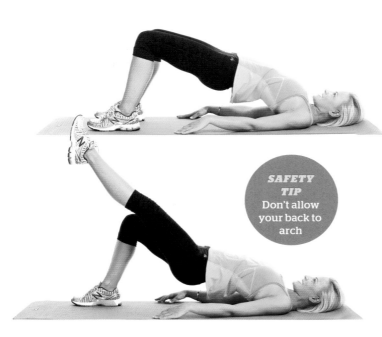

SAFETY TIP
Don't allow your back to arch

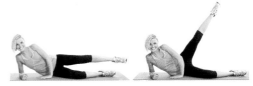

Leg raises
Area trained: Bottom

» Lie on your side with your upper body supported by your elbow, lower leg bent and upper leg straight.
» Lift your upper leg slightly off the floor – this is your starting position.
» Raise your upper leg to 45 degrees, then slowly lower back to the start and repeat.
» Turn onto the other side and repeat with the other leg halfway through each set.

Wall sit
Area trained: Front thighs

» Place a stability ball against a wall and rest against it, facing away from the wall so your lower back is supported and your hips and knees are bent to 90 degrees.
» Hold this position for the allotted time.

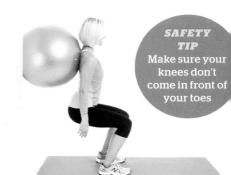

SAFETY TIP
Make sure your knees don't come in front of your toes

14-day drop a dress size diet plan

🕐 **7.30am** Breakfast
» 1 morning refresher juice (p120)
» Supplements

🕐 **10.30am** Snack
» 1 apple and 1 tablespoon of mixed raw nuts and/or seeds

🕐 **1pm** Lunch
» Tandoori chicken salad (p124)

🕐 **4pm** Snack
» 1 small fat-free Greek yoghurt with half a pack of berries

🕐 **7pm** Dinner
» Cod with stir-fried vegetables (p130)

Day 7

14-day drop a dress size workout plan

🕐 **Rest day**, all levels

14-day drop a dress size diet plan

🕐 **7am** Lemon cleanse
» 1 glass of room-temperature water with a squeeze of lemon

🕐 **7.30am** Breakfast
» 1 beetroot liver cleanse juice (p120)
» Supplements

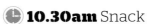
Day 8

🕐 **10.30am** Snack
» 1 apple and 2 tablespoons of mixed raw nuts and/or seeds

🕐 **1pm** Lunch
» Green goddess soup (p122)

🕐 **4pm** Snack
» 2 tablespoons of mixed raw nuts and/or seeds and 2 handfuls of blueberries

🕐 **7pm** Dinner
» Cauliflower detox soup (p122)

🕐 **10pm** Overnight detox drink
» 1 cup of instant miso soup

14-day **drop a dress size workout plan**

🕐 **5pm** 45 mins cardio or any class, all levels

🕐 **6pm** Core and tummy toning session

Complete the following circuit:

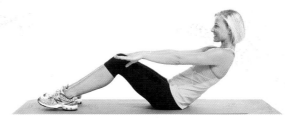

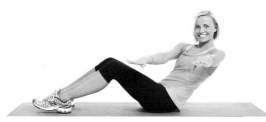

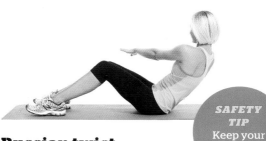

Twisting crunch
Areas trained:
Upper and lower stomach, sides of stomach

» Lie on your back with your feet flat on the floor, hips and knees bent, hands at your temples.
» Slowly lift your shoulders off the floor and twist your upper body to the left, taking your right shoulder towards your left knee while drawing your left knee towards your elbow.
» Lower back down and repeat the move, twisting to the right.

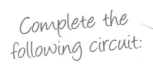

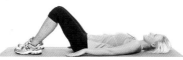

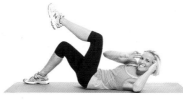

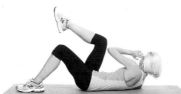

SAFETY TIP
Keep your lower back in contact with the floor

Beginner	Intermediate	Advanced
2 sets of 10 reps	2 sets of 16 reps	3 sets of 16-20 reps
5 twists each side	**8 twists each side**	**8-10 twists each side**

Russian twist
Areas trained: Upper stomach, sides of stomach

» Sit on the floor with your hips and knees bent and your arms straight out in front of you. Lean back to 45 degrees.
» Twist to the left and pause, return to the centre and twist to the right to complete one rep. Repeat for half of the prescribed reps.
» Lower your torso slightly further, twisting to the right, and then left to complete one set.

SAFETY TIP
Keep your back straight

Beginner	Intermediate	Advanced
2 sets of **6-8 reps**	2 sets of **8-10 reps**	2 sets of **10-12 reps**

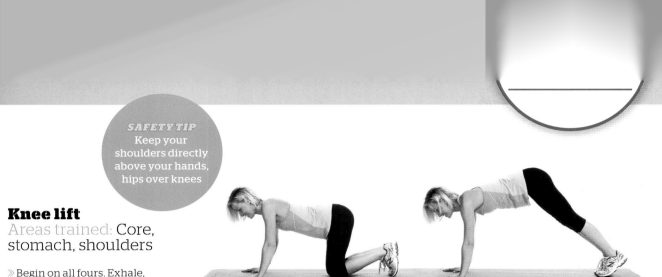

SAFETY TIP
Keep your shoulders directly above your hands, hips over knees

Knee lift
Areas trained: Core, stomach, shoulders

» Begin on all fours. Exhale, tightening your abs and engaging your pelvic floor muscles, lifting your knees off the floor and holding for the allotted time.
» Lower slowly and repeat.

Beginner	Intermediate	Advanced
2 sets of **10 reps** (1-sec hold)	2 sets of **10 reps** (2-sec hold)	2 sets of **10 reps** (3-sec hold)

Hip bridge
Areas trained: Core, stomach, bottom

» Lie flat on your back with knees bent and feet flat on the floor, your arms by your sides.
» Tighten your stomach and engage your pelvic floor muscles, lifting your hips to form a straight line from your shoulders to your knees.
» Hold for a two-count, lower and repeat..

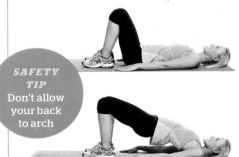

SAFETY TIP
Don't allow your back to arch

Reverse crunch
Area trained: Lower stomach

» Lie on your back with your feet off the floor, hips and knees bent at 90 degrees, thighs pressed together, and arms by your sides.
» Raise your hips off the floor towards your ribs, concentrating on using your lower stomach to create the movement.
» Lower back to the starting position, allowing your hips to lightly touch the floor and repeat.

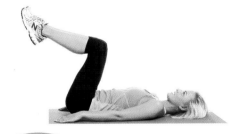

SAFETY TIP
Keep your neck and arms relaxed throughout and perform the movement slowly and under control

Beginner	Intermediate	Advanced
2 sets of **8-12 reps**	3 sets of **10-12 reps**	3 sets of **12-15 reps**

Beginner	Intermediate	Advanced
2 sets of **8-10 reps**	2 sets of **10-12 reps**	2 sets of **12-15 reps**

14-day drop a dress size diet plan

🕐 **7am** Lemon cleanse
» 1 glass of room-temperature water with a squeeze of lemon

🕐 **7.30am** Breakfast
» 1 breakfast boost juice (p121)
» Supplements

🕐 **10.30am** Snack
» 1 apple and 2 tablespoons of mixed raw nuts and/or seeds

🕐 **1pm** Lunch
» Carrot soup (p123)

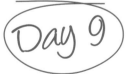

🕐 **4pm** Snack
» 2 tablespoons of mixed raw nuts and/or seeds and 2 handfuls of blueberries

🕐 **7pm** Dinner
» Lovely lettuce soup (p122)

🕐 **10pm** Overnight detox drink
» 1 cup of instant miso soup

14-day drop a dress size workout plan

🕐 **5pm** Complete the following circuit:

Beginner: 30 secs each exercise, repeat 4 times

Intermediate: 45 secs each exercise, repeat 4 times

Advanced: 60 secs each exercise, repeat 4 times

Jumping lunges
Areas trained: Thighs, bottom

» Begin standing with one foot in front of the other, then bend your knees and lower into a lunge.
» Quickly jump up and switch legs in mid-air, then lunge down and repeat for the allotted time.

SAFETY TIP
Make sure your front knee stays behind your toes and above your ankle

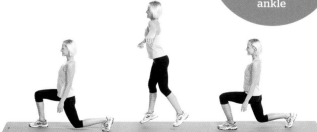

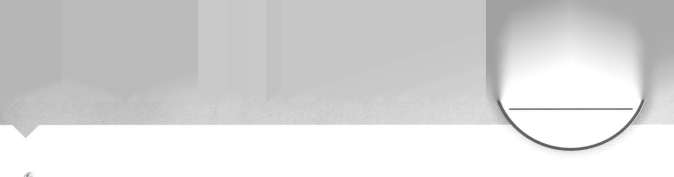

Scissors
Area trained: Lower stomach

» Lie on your back with your arms on the floor by your sides, legs outstretched at a height you can hold without arching your back.
» Take your left leg over your right so they cross, then apart, then bring your right leg over your left.
» Continue crossing your legs for the allotted time.

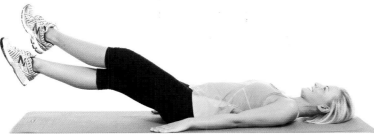

SAFETY TIP
Keep your lower back in contact with the floor

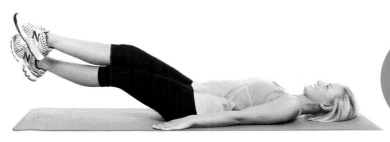

SAFETY TIP
Keep your abs tight, focusing on drawing your belly button to your spine. Don't allow your hips to sag or your back to arch

Explosive push-up
Areas trained: Chest, shoulders, rear upper arms

» Begin in a box or modified push-up position, hands slightly wider than shoulder-width apart.
» Lower your chest to just above the floor.
» As quickly and powerfully as you can, push through your hands, straightening your arms and taking your hands off the floor momentarily.
» Place your hands back on the floor and repeat the move for the allotted time.
» To increase the challenge, clap your hands together when they leave the floor.

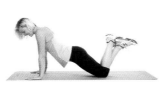
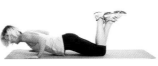
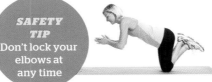

SAFETY TIP
Don't lock your elbows at any time

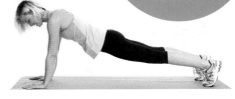

Plank
Areas trained: Abs, lower back

» Begin on all fours then tighten your stomach and walk your feet back into plank position. Your body should form a straight line from head to toes.
» Hold this position for the allotted time.

Push-up burpees

Areas trained: Cardio, thighs, bottom, chest, shoulders, rear upper arms, stomach

>> Begin in plank position, shoulders over your hands, tummy tight and your body in a straight line.
>> Lower your chest to the floor, performing a push-up. Straighten your arms and return to plank position.
>> Jump your feet towards your hands, then jump straight up, taking your arms up.
>> Land softly and squat down, placing your hands either side of your feet, then jump your feet back into plank position. This is one rep. Repeat to complete the set.

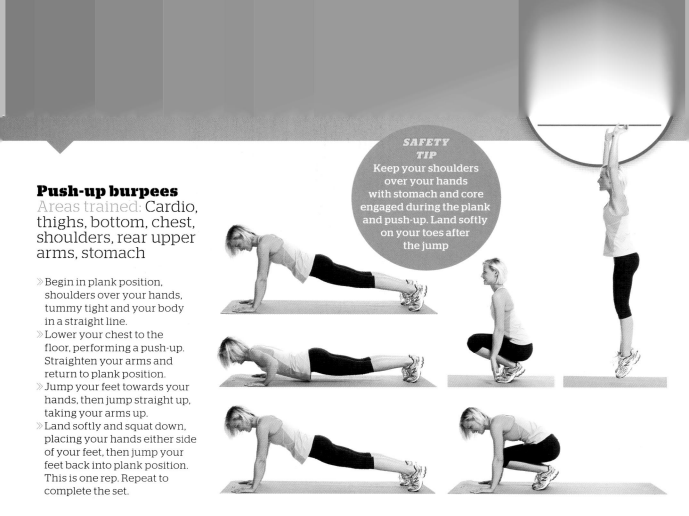

SAFETY TIP
Keep your shoulders over your hands with stomach and core engaged during the plank and push-up. Land softly on your toes after the jump

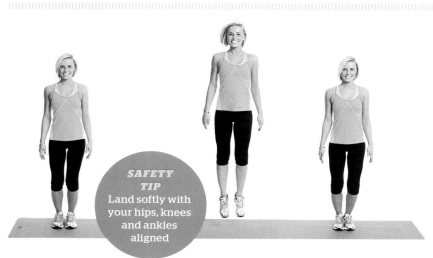

SAFETY TIP
Land softly with your hips, knees and ankles aligned

Side jumps

Areas trained: Thighs, calves

>> Stand to one side of an imaginary line. Jump with both feet over to the other side, then immediately back again. Continue for the allotted time.

Plus

>> Running or swimming

Beginner	Intermediate	Advanced
30 mins	40 mins	50 mins

14-day **drop a dress size diet plan**

🕐 **7.30am** Breakfast
» 1 vitamin vitality juice (p120)
» Supplements

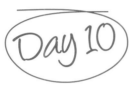

🕐 **10.30am** Snack
» 1 apple and 1 tablespoon of mixed raw nuts and/or seeds

🕐 **1pm** Lunch
» Salmon fillet salad (p130)

🕐 **4pm** Snack
» 1 small fat-free Greek yoghurt with half a pack of berries

🕐 **7pm** Dinner
» Ratatouille with 1 small baked sweet potato (p125)

14-day **drop a dress size workout plan**

🕐 **5pm** 1-hour Pilates class or DVD, all levels

14-day **drop a dress size diet plan**

🕐 **7.30am** Breakfast
» 1 green pineapple juice (p120)
» Supplements

🕐 **10.30am** Snack
» 1 apple and 1 tablespoon of mixed raw nuts and/or seeds

🕐 **1pm** Lunch
» Tuna Niçoise salad (p124)

🕐 **4pm** Snack
» 1 small fat-free Greek yoghurt with half a pack of berries

🕐 **7pm** Dinner
» Falafel (p128) with cauliflower 'couscous' (p126) and beetroot dip (p124)

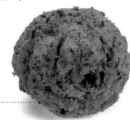

14-day **drop a dress size workout plan**

🕐 **5pm** Interval training

Beginner	Intermediate	Advanced
1-min walk	2-min jog	1-min jog
1-min jog	1-min sprint	2-min run
x15	**x10**	**x10**

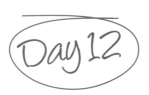
Day 12

14-day drop a dress size workout plan

🕐 **Rest day**, all levels

14-day drop a dress size diet plan

🕐 **7.30am** Breakfast
» 1 tomato and celery juice (p120)
» Supplements

🕐 **10.30am** Snack
» 1 apple and 1 tablespoon of raw nuts and/or seeds

🕐 **1pm** Lunch
» Cottage cheese salad (p128)

🕐 **4pm** Snack
» 1 small fat-free Greek yoghurt with half a pack of berries

🕐 **7pm** Dinner
» Lentil soup (p130)

14-day drop a dress size diet plan

🕐 **7.30am** Breakfast
» 1 morning refresher juice (p120)
» Supplements

🕐 **10.30am** Snack
» 1 apple and 1 tablespoon of mixed raw nuts and/or seeds

🕐 **1pm** Lunch
» Salmon fillet salad (p130)

🕐 **4pm** Snack
» 1 small fat-free Greek yoghurt with half a pack of berries

🕐 **7pm** Dinner
» Roast pork with Puy lentils (p128)

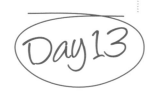
Day 13

14-day drop a dress size workout plan

🕐 **9am** 1-hour cardio or class, all levels

🕐 **10am** Lower-body toning session
Repeat circuit from day 6 (p78)

14-day **drop a dress size diet plan**

🕐 **7.30am** Breakfast
≫ 1 breakfast boost
juice (p121)
≫ Supplements

🕐 **10.30am** Snack
≫ 1 apple and 1 tablespoon
of mixed raw nuts
and/or seeds

🕐 **1pm** Lunch
≫ Feta and mint
salad (p124)

🕐 **4pm** Snack
≫ 1 small fat-free Greek
yoghurt with half a pack
of berries

🕐 **7pm** Dinner
≫ Grilled pollock with
salsa verde and butter
bean mash (p127)

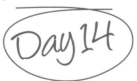
Day 14

14-day **drop a dress size workout plan**

🕐 **9am** Interval training

Beginner	Intermediate	Advanced
1-min walk	2-min jog	1-min jog
1-min jog	1-min sprint	2-min run
x15	**x10**	1-min sprint
		x10

🕐 **10am** Core and tummy
toning session
Repeat circuit from
day 8 (p82)

≫

Your results

Track your progress on the 14-day bootcamp

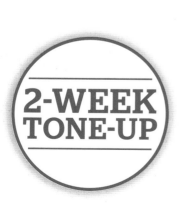	Before	After 1 week	After 2 weeks
Weight			
Arms			
Bust			
Waist			
Hips			
Thighs			

2-WEEK TONE-UP

Well done on a great result!

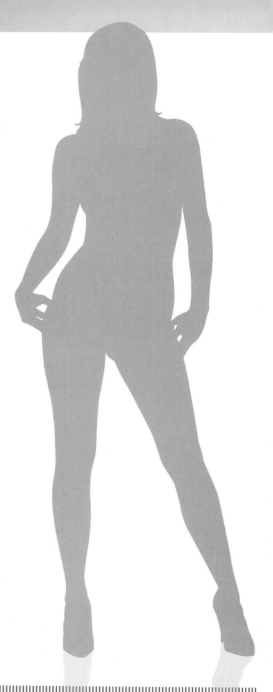

4-week

total body blitz plan

Overhaul your body in one month!

Get ready to work hard and reap the rewards. This plan will help you transform your figure

Be sure to fill in your vital statistics on page 118, so you can measure your results

Caution: As with any diet, you should consult your doctor before starting this plan and if you experience any unpleasant symptoms you should stop the diet and see a healthcare professional immediately. This plan is not suitable for those who are underweight, pregnant or planning on becoming pregnant, or breastfeeding. This plan should not be followed for more than one month.

Things to remember

You can lose up to a stone on this healthy four-week plan. What are you waiting for?

Equipment you'll need
» Juicer to juice fruit and vegetables
» Blender or hand blender for soups

» This is the big one, and after four weeks on this plan you should have shifted a serious amount of weight. How much will depend on how strictly you stick to it and how hard you work out, but between 10lb to a stone is achievable! Like the other bootcamp plans in this book, the 4-week total body blitz starts with a short, sharp detox. Then you'll mix up higher and lower-calorie days to keep shocking your body so it doesn't plateau. On this plan you also begin reintroducing starches and beans in the latter weeks, and there's plenty of protein to help replenish and restore your metabolism-boosting muscles.

The rules

» On detox days, you start with a glass of water with a squeeze of lemon juice. Then breakfast is a juice, and lunch and dinner are soups. The morning and afternoon snacks are two tablespoons of mixed raw nuts or seeds and fruit. The day ends with an overnight detox drink, which is a light miso soup.

» For the remaining part of the first week, you add in protein with your lunchtime salad and a cooked dinner. When the plan says salad you can eat unlimited amounts of salad leaves and non-root vegetables but you must limit the salad dressing to one or two tablespoons. Your morning snack is a piece of fruit and mixed raw nuts and/or seeds and your afternoon snack is fat-free Greek yoghurt and berries.

» In the remaining three weeks of this plan, you start each week with a one-day detox, then you can eat protein, salad and veggies and gradually reintroduce some carbs such as wholegrains and beans to your diet.

» On non-detox days if you need post-workout replenishment to aid your recovery, have a protein bar or shake.

» Aim to drink 1.5 litres of water a day.

» Take the following supplements every morning with your breakfast:
» Multivitamin/mineral
» Omega-3
» Mixed antioxidants

» Exercise and relax. Follow the exercise plan for each day and aim to sleep at least seven hours a night.

» Don't drink coffee, tea, cola or other caffeinated drinks, including green tea. Replace them with water, or herbal teas and decaf coffee without milk.

» Don't drink alcohol of any kind. Don't drink fruit juice, smoothies or fruit cordials. The only juices you should drink are those you have made according to the recipes on the plan.

» Don't eat any starchy carbs such as white bread, pasta and rice, potatoes, cakes and biscuits. And no chocolate!

4-week total body blitz diet plan

🕐 **7am** Lemon cleanse
» 1 glass of room-temperature water with a squeeze of lemon

🕐 **7.30am** Breakfast
» 1 beetroot liver cleanse juice (p120)
» Supplements

🕐 **10.30am** Snack
» 1 apple and 2 tablespoons of mixed raw nuts and/or seeds (Brazil nuts, walnuts, almonds, pumpkin and sunflower seeds)

🕐 **1pm** Lunch
» Green goddess soup (p123)

🕐 **4pm** Snack
» 2 tablespoons of mixed raw nuts and/or seeds and 2 handfuls of blueberries

🕐 **7pm** Dinner
» Cauliflower detox soup (p122)

🕐 **10pm** Overnight detox drink
» 1 cup of instant miso soup

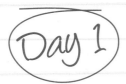

Day 1

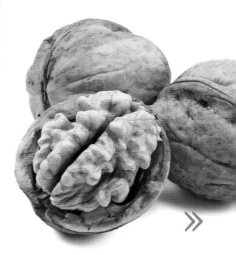

4-week total body blitz workout plan

Kit you'll need
» 2 x 4-8kg dumbbells
» 2 x 3-5kg dumbbells
» 5-8kg medicine ball
» Resistance band
» Stability ball
» Step
» Skipping rope

🕐 **9am** Upper-body toning session

Find your level

Beginner: Choose 5 exercises and complete 2 circuits, performing each exercise for 30 secs

Intermediate: Choose 7 exercises and complete 2 circuits, performing each exercise for 45 secs

Advanced: Complete 2 circuits of all exercises, performing each exercise for 1 min

Incline push-up
Areas trained: Upper chest, shoulders, rear upper arms

» Begin in a full or modified push-up position with your hands just wider than shoulder-width apart and your feet on a step or box.
» Bend your elbows and lower your chest to an inch above the ground, keeping your body in a straight line.
» Push through your hands, straightening your arms to return to the start position. Repeat.

SAFETY TIP
Keep your abs tight and don't let your hips sag

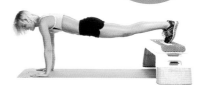
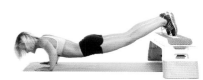

Extra wide push-up
Areas trained: Chest, shoulders, rear upper arms

» Begin in a full or modified push-up position with your body in a straight line, hands under your shoulders and your arms around three inches wider than they would be for a regular push-up.
» Slowly and with control, lower your chest to just above the floor, then straighten your arms to return to the start. Repeat.

SAFETY TIP
Don't allow your hips to sag

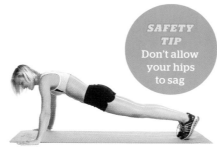
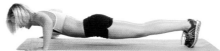

Plank transfer
Areas trained: Shoulders, core, rear upper arms

» Begin in plank position, upper body resting on your forearms, your stomach tight and body in a straight line from feet to shoulders.

» Transfer your weight slightly to your right side, straightening your left arm, placing your hand on the floor under your shoulder. Repeat with your right arm to come into a full push-up position.

» Hold for a count of one then return to resting on your forearms, one arm at a time to complete one rep. Repeat, starting with your right arm.

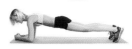
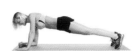
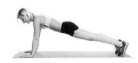

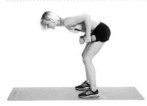
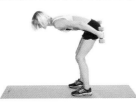

Tricep kickbacks
Area trained: Rear upper arms

» Stand with feet hip-width apart, holding a 3-5kg dumbbell in each hand by your sides.

» Bend forwards 90 degrees from the hips, keeping your back straight, bending your elbows to 90 degrees so your forearms point towards the floor, your upper arms against your sides. This is your starting position.

» Extend your arms so your hands are just past your hips.

» Return to the start position and repeat, keeping your upper arms still.

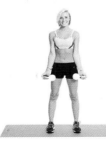
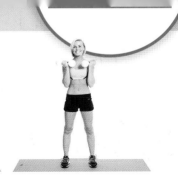

Bicep curl
Area trained: Front upper arms

» Stand with your feet shoulder-width apart holding a 4-8kg dumbbell in each hand, with arms by your sides, palms facing forward.

» Bend your elbows, taking the dumbbells up towards your shoulders, keeping your elbows touching your sides with upper arms still.

» Lower the dumbbells down to the start and repeat.

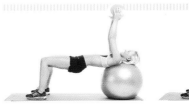
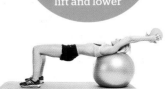

Medicine ball pull-over
Areas trained: Chest, shoulders, upper back

» Lie back on a stability ball, holding a 5-8kg medicine ball with hands shoulder-width apart, and walk your feet forward until only your head and upper back are supported, with your knees bent at 90 degrees.

» Keeping your stomach tight, lift the medicine ball until it's directly over your chest, keeping your arms straight – this is your starting position.

» Slowly extend your arms straight behind you, in line with your body, with upper arms close to your ears.

» Slowly raise your arms to the starting position and repeat the move.

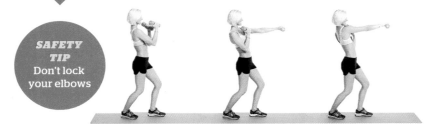

SAFETY TIP
Don't lock your elbows

Shadow boxing
Areas trained: Shoulders, arms

» Stand with your left foot in front of your right and your left shoulder slightly in front of your right.
» Quickly punch straight ahead with your left hand, bringing it back

and then repeating with your right hand. Continue for the allotted time for your level.
» Hold a dumbbell in each hand to increase the difficulty if required.

High row
Area trained: Upper back

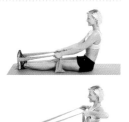

» Begin seated with your legs straight out in front of you and a resistance band wrapped around your feet, holding an end in each hand. There should be a little tension in the band at this point.
» Bring your hands towards your shoulders, taking your elbows up and out so they are level with your shoulders. Return to the start and repeat.

Upright row
Areas trained: Shoulders, upper back

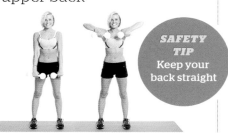

» Begin standing with feet hip-width apart, holding a 4-8kg dumbbell in each hand with your hands by your thighs.
» Bring your hands up towards your shoulders, taking your elbows upwards and outwards.
» Slowly straighten your arms and return to the start. Repeat.

SAFETY TIP
Keep your back straight

Tricep dips
Areas trained: Rear upper arms, shoulders

» Begin seated on a chair, placing your hands just outside your thighs. Walk your feet forward, coming off the chair so your body weight is supported by your hands and feet.
» Lift your left foot off the floor and straighten your knee.
» Lower yourself towards the floor so your elbows are bent at 90 degrees, push through your hands to straighten your arms and repeat.
» Continue for the allotted time, changing feet halfway through.

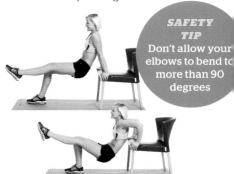

SAFETY TIP
Don't allow your elbows to bend to more than 90 degrees

Plus
» Skipping workout

Beginner	Intermediate	Advanced
Skip 30 secs	Skip 40 secs	Skip 45 secs
March on the spot 30 secs	March on the spot 20 secs	March on the spot 15 secs
x12	x12	x12

4-week total body blitz diet plan

🕐 **7am** Lemon cleanse
» 1 glass of room-temperature water with a squeeze of lemon

🕐 **7.30am** Breakfast
» 1 breakfast boost juice (p121)
» Supplements

Day 2

🕐 **10.30am** Snack
» 1 apple and 2 tablespoons of mixed raw nuts or seeds

🕐 **1pm** Lunch
» Carrot soup (p123)

🕐 **4pm** Snack
» 2 tablespoons of mixed raw nuts or seeds and 2 handfuls of blueberries

🕐 **7pm** Dinner
» Lovely lettuce soup (p122)

🕐 **10pm** Overnight detox drink
» 1 cup of instant miso soup

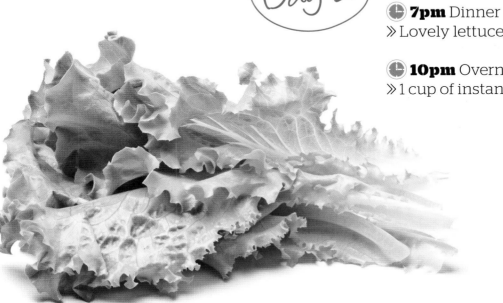

»

4-week total body blitz workout plan

🕕 **6pm** Core and tummy toning session

Twisting crunch
Area trained: Stomach

Complete the following circuit:

» Lie on your back with your feet flat on the floor, hips and knees bent, hands lightly touching your temples.
» Slowly lift your shoulders off the floor and twist your upper body to the left, taking your right shoulder towards your left knee, while simultaneously drawing your left knee in towards your elbow.
» Lower yourself back down slowly and repeat the move, twisting to the right.

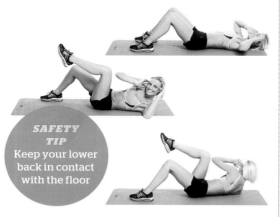

Beginner	Intermediate	Advanced
2 sets of 10 reps	2 sets of 16 reps	3 sets of 16-20 reps
5 twists each side	**8 twists each side**	**8-10 twists each side**

Reverse crunch
Area trained: Lower stomach

» Lie on your back with your feet off the floor, hips and knees bent at 90 degrees, thighs pressed together, arms by your sides.
» Raise your hips off the floor towards your ribs, concentrating on using your lower stomach to create the movement.
» Lower your body back to the starting position, allowing your hips to lightly touch the floor, then repeat.

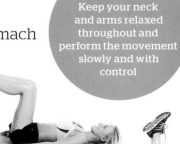

Beginner	Intermediate	Advanced
2 sets of	3 sets of	3 sets of
8-12 reps	**10-12 reps**	**12-15 reps**

Knee lift
Areas trained: Core, stomach, shoulders

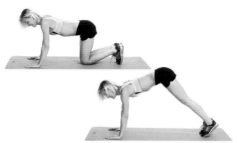

» Begin on all fours. Exhale, tightening your tummy and engaging your pelvic floor muscles, lifting your knees off the floor and holding for the allotted time for your level.
» Lower slowly to the floor and repeat.

Beginner	Intermediate	Advanced
2 sets of 10 reps	2 set of 10 reps	2 sets of 10 reps
1-sec hold	**2-sec hold**	**3-sec hold**

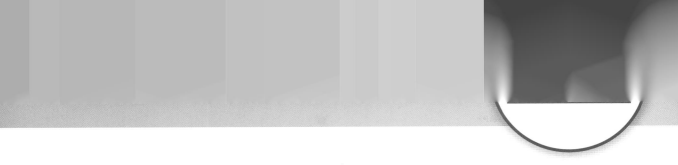

Russian twist
Areas trained: Upper stomach, sides of stomach

» Sit on the floor with your hips and knees bent and your arms straight out in front of you. Lean back to 45 degrees.

» Twist to the left and pause,

return to the centre and twist to the right to complete one rep. Repeat for half of the prescribed reps.

» Lower your torso slightly further, twisting to the right, and then to the left to complete one set.

SAFETY TIP
Keep your back straight

Beginner	Intermediate	Advanced
2 sets of **6-8 reps**	2 sets of **8-10 reps**	2 sets of **10-12 reps**

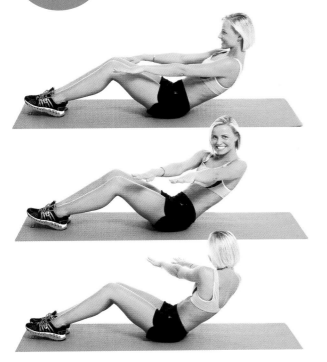

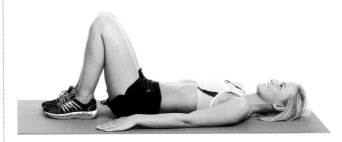

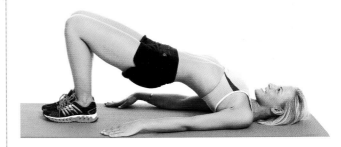

Hip bridge
Areas trained: Core, stomach, bottom

SAFETY TIP
Don't allow your back to arch

» Lie flat on your back with knees bent and feet flat on the floor, arms by your sides.

» Tighten your stomach and engage your pelvic floor muscles, lifting your hips to form a straight line from your shoulders to your knees.

» Hold for a count of two, lower your body and repeat.

Beginner	Intermediate	Advanced
2 sets of **8-10 reps**	2 sets of **10-12 reps**	2 sets of **12-15 reps**

»

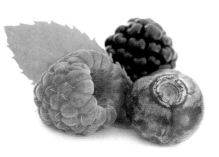

4-week **total body blitz workout plan**

🕐 **Rest day**, all levels

4-week **total body blitz diet plan**

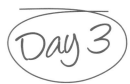
Day 3

🕐 **7.30am** Breakfast
» 1 vitamin vitality juice (p120)
» Supplements

🕐 **10.30am** Snack
» 1 apple and 1 tablespoon of mixed raw nuts and/or seeds

🕐 **1pm** Lunch
» Tandoori chicken salad (p124)

🕐 **4pm** Snack
» 1 small fat-free Greek yoghurt with half a pack of berries

🕐 **7pm** Dinner
» Stuffed mushrooms (p128)

4-week **total body blitz diet plan**

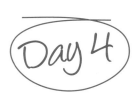
Day 4

🕐 **7.30am** Breakfast
» 1 sunrise juice (p120)
» Supplements

🕐 **10.30am** Snack
» 1 apple and 1 tablespoon of mixed raw nuts and/or seeds

🕐 **1pm** Lunch

» Feta and mint salad (p124)

🕐 **4pm** Snack
» 1 small fat-free Greek yoghurt with half a pack of berries

🕐 **7pm** Dinner
» Cauliflower pizza (p126)

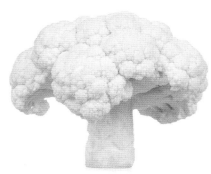

4-week total body blitz workout plan

⏰ 8am Interval training

Beginner	Intermediate	Advanced
1-min walk	2-min jog	1-min jog
1-min jog	1-min sprint	2-min run
x15	**x10**	**x10**

⏰ 8.30am Lower-body toning

Beginner: Choose 4 exercises and complete 2 circuits, performing each exercise for 30 secs

Intermediate: Choose 5 exercises and complete 2 circuits, performing each exercise for 45 secs

Advanced: Complete 2 circuits of all exercises, performing each exercise for 1 min

Walking lunges
Areas trained: Thighs, bottom

» Stand with feet hip-width apart holding a dumbbell or a bottle of water in each hand above your head with arms straight and hands slightly wider than shoulder-width apart.
» Take a large step forward with your right foot then lunge down, bending both knees and lowering down until your back knee is just above the floor.
» Straighten your legs and take a large step forward with your left foot and repeat. Continue alternating legs.

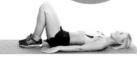

SAFETY TIP
Don't allow your back to arch

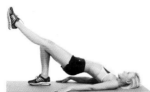

Donkey kicks
Areas trained: Bottom, rear thighs

» Begin on all fours then extend your right leg out behind you, slightly off the floor.
» Raise your leg, keeping it straight so your foot is just higher than your hips, squeezing your bottom as you do so.
» Lower to just above the ground and repeat the move.
» Change legs halfway through each set.

Bridge
Areas trained: Bottom, core

» Lie on your back with your knees bent, feet flat on the floor and your arms by your sides.
» Tighten your stomach and lift your hips off the floor into a bridge position with your body in a straight line.
» Straighten your left leg, keeping your hips level. Hold, then lower your body back down and repeat.
» Change legs halfway through each set.

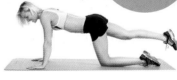

SAFETY TIP
Keep your back straight

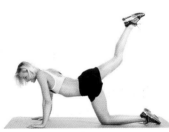

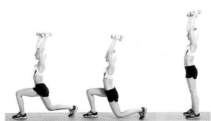

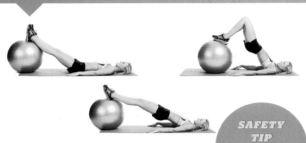

Stability ball leg curl
Areas trained: Rear thighs, bottom, lower back

SAFETY TIP
Keep your back straight

» Begin lying on your back, feet resting on a stability ball, arms by your sides for support.
» Lift your hips to form a straight line between your feet and shoulders.

» Maintaining this position, bend your knees to roll the ball towards you.
» Slowly straighten your knees and lower your hips to the floor, then repeat the move.

Jump squat
Areas trained: Front thighs, bottom

» Stand with your feet shoulder-width apart, hands on your hips.
» Bend your hips and knees and squat down as if you were going to sit on a chair behind you, taking care not to lean too far forward from the hips.

» Quickly straighten your legs, jumping as high as you can, landing softly then returning to the start position. Repeat.

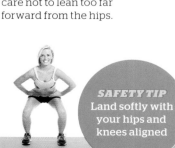

SAFETY TIP
Land softly with your hips and knees aligned

Squat thrusts
Areas trained: Inner, outer and front thighs, bottom, shoulders, core

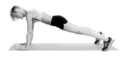

» Start in plank position with your shoulders over your hands, tummy tight and body in a straight line from shoulders to feet.
» Jump your feet out to the sides and back together, then jump your feet forward towards your hands.
» Jump your feet back and repeat.

SAFETY TIP
Keep the knee of the straight leg soft, and not locked

Leg raises
Area trained: Bottom

» Lie on your side with your upper body supported by your elbow, lower leg bent and upper leg straight.
» Lift your upper leg slightly off the floor – this is your starting position.
» Raise your upper leg to 45 degrees, then lower back and repeat.
» Turn onto the other side and repeat with the other leg halfway through each set.

Wall sit
Area trained: Front thighs

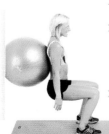

» Place a stability ball against a wall and rest against it, facing away from the wall so your lower back is supported and your hips and knees are bent to 90 degrees.
» Hold this position for the allotted time.

SAFETY TIP
Make sure your knees don't come in front of your toes

4-week total body blitz diet plan

7.30am Breakfast
» 1 green pineapple juice (p120)
» Supplements

10.30am Snack
» 1 apple and 1 tablespoon of mixed raw nuts and/or seeds

1pm Lunch
» Tuna Niçoise salad (p124)

4pm Snack
» 1 small fat-free Greek yoghurt with half a pack of berries

7pm Dinner
» California omelette (p126)

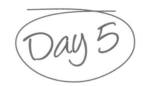

Day 5

4-week total body blitz workout plan

9am 1-hour class or DVD, all levels

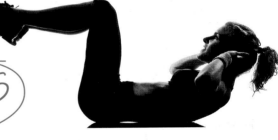

4-week total body blitz diet plan

7.30am Breakfast
» 1 tomato and celery juice (p120)
» Supplements

10.30am Snack
» 1 apple and 1 tablespoon of mixed raw nuts and/or seeds

1pm Lunch
» Cottage cheese salad (p128)

Day 6

4pm Snack
» 1 small fat-free Greek yoghurt with half a pack of berries

7pm Dinner
» Chicken stir-fry (p126)

4-week total body blitz workout plan

🕕 **6pm** Fat-burning circuit:

Beginner: 30 secs each exercise, repeat 4 times

Intermediate: 45 secs each exercise, repeat 4 times

Advanced: 60 secs each exercise, repeat 4 times

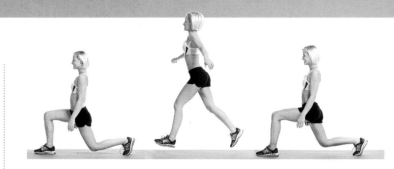

Side jumps
Areas trained: Thighs, calves

» Stand to one side of an imaginary line. Jump with both feet over to the other side, then immediately back again. Continue for the allotted time.

SAFETY TIP
Land softly with your hips, knees and ankles aligned

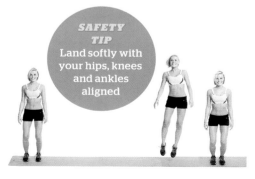

Jumping lunges
Areas trained: Thighs, bottom

» Begin standing with one foot in front of the other, then bend your knees and lower into a lunge.

» Quickly jump up and switch legs in mid-air, then lunge down and repeat for the allotted time.

SAFETY TIP
Make sure your front knee stays behind your toes and directly above your ankle

Scissors
Area trained: Lower stomach

» Lie on your back with your arms on the floor by your sides, legs outstretched at a height you can hold without arching your back.

» Take your left leg over your right so they cross, then bring your right leg over your left.

» Continue crossing your legs for the allotted time.

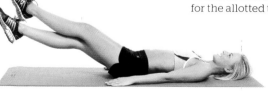

SAFETY TIP
Keep your lower back in contact with the floor

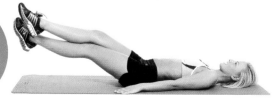

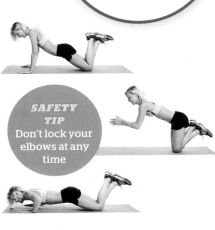

Plank
Areas trained: Abs, lower back

» Begin on all fours then tighten your stomach and walk your feet back into plank position. Your body should form a straight line from head to toes.
» Hold this position for the allotted time.

SAFETY TIP
Keep your abs tight, focusing on drawing your belly button to your spine. Don't allow your hips to sag or your back to arch

SAFETY TIP
Don't lock your elbows at any time

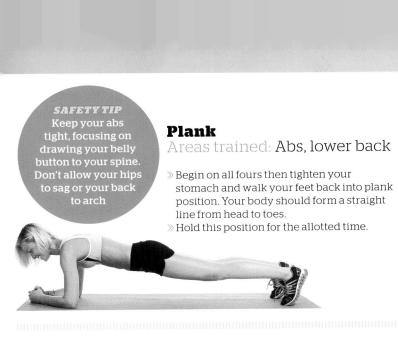

Push-up burpees
Areas trained: Cardio, thighs, bottom, chest, shoulders, rear upper arms, stomach

» Begin in plank position, shoulders over your hands and tummy tight.

» Lower your chest to the floor, performing a push-up. Straighten your arms and return to plank position.
» Jump your feet towards your hands, then jump straight up, taking your arms up.
» Land softly and squat down, placing your hands either side of your feet, then jump your feet back into plank position. This is one rep. Repeat for the allotted time.

SAFETY TIP
Keep your shoulders over your hands with stomach engaged during the plank and push-up. Land softly on your toes after the jump

Explosive push-up
Areas trained: Chest, shoulders, rear upper arms

» Begin in a full or modified push-up position, hands slightly wider than shoulder-width apart.
» Lower your chest to just above the floor.
» As quickly and powerfully as you can, push through your hands, straightening your arms and taking your hands off the floor momentarily.
» Place your hands back on the floor and repeat the move for the allotted time.
» To increase the challenge, clap your hands together when they leave the floor.

Plus
» Running intervals

Beginner	Intermediate	Advanced
1-min walk	2-min jog	1-min jog
1-min jog	1-min sprint	1-min run
x15	**x10**	1-min sprint
		x10

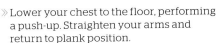

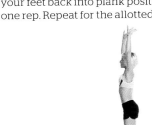

4-week total body blitz diet plan

🕐 **7.30am** Breakfast
» 1 morning refresher juice (p120)
» Supplements

🕐 **10.30am** Snack
» 1 apple and 1 tablespoon of mixed raw nuts and/or seeds

🕐 **1pm** Lunch
» Egg salad (p127) with tofu mayonnaise (p126)

🕐 **4pm** Snack
» 1 small fat-free Greek yoghurt with half a pack of berries

🕐 **7pm** Dinner
» Prawn skewers (p127) with cauliflower 'couscous' (p126)

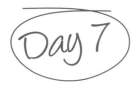
Day 7

4-week total body blitz workout plan

🕐 **9am** 1-hour Pilates class or DVD, all levels

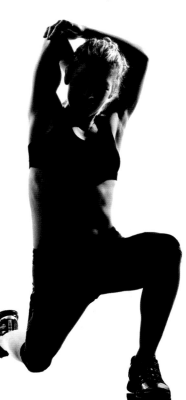

4-week total body blitz diet plan

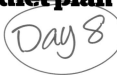
Day 8

week 2

🕐 **7am** Lemon cleanse
» 1 glass of room-temperature water with a squeeze of lemon

🕐 **7.30am** Breakfast
» 1 beetroot liver cleanse juice (p120)
» Supplements

🕐 **10.30am** Snack
» 1 apple and 2 tablespoons of mixed raw nuts or seeds

🕐 **1pm** Lunch
» Green goddess soup (p122)

🕐 **4pm** Snack
» 2 tablespoons of mixed raw nuts or seeds and a handful of blueberries

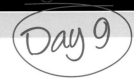
7pm Dinner
» Cauliflower detox soup (p122)

10pm Overnight detox drink
» 1 cup of instant miso soup

4-week total body blitz workout plan

8am Skipping workout

Beginner	Intermediate	Advanced
Skip 30 secs	Skip 40 secs	Skip 45 secs
March on the spot 30 secs	March on the spot 20 secs	March on the spot 15 secs
x14	x14	x14

Plus

» Repeat day 1 upper-body circuit (p94)

Reps and sets:

Beginner:
Choose 5 of the 10 exercises and complete 2 circuits, performing each exercise for 35 secs

Intermediate:
Choose 7 exercises and complete 2

circuits, performing each exercise for 50 secs

Advanced:
Complete all exercises and complete 2 circuits, performing each exercise for 70 secs

4-week total body blitz diet plan

7am Lemon cleanse
» 1 glass of room-temperature water with a squeeze of lemon

7.30am Breakfast
» 1 breakfast boost juice (p121)
» Supplements

10.30am Snack
» 1 apple and 2 tablespoons of raw nuts or seeds

1pm Lunch
» Cottage cheese salad (p128)

4pm Snack
» 2 tablespoons mixed raw nuts and/or seeds and 2 handfuls of blueberries

7pm Dinner
» Roast pollock with salsa verde and butter bean mash (p127)

4-week workout plan

8am Core and tummy toning session

» Repeat day 2 circuit (p98)

Reps and sets:

Twisting crunch
Beginner:
2 sets of 12 (6 twists each side)
Intermediate:
2 sets of 14 (7 twists each side)
Advanced:
3 sets of 18 (9 twists each side)

Knee lift
Beginner:
2 sets of 12 (1-sec hold)
Intermediate:
2 set of 12 (2-sec hold)
Advanced:
2 sets of 12 (3-sec hold)

Russian twist
Beginner:
2 sets of 8
Intermediate:
2 sets of 10
Advanced:
2 sets of 12-15

Reverse crunch
Beginner:
2 sets of 10
Intermediate:
3 sets of 12
Advanced:
3 sets of 15

Hip bridge
Beginner:
2 sets of 10
Intermediate:
2 sets of 12
Advanced:
2 sets of 15

4-week total body blitz diet plan

🕐 **7.30am** Breakfast
» 1 vitamin vitality juice (p120)
» Supplements

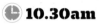 *Day 10*

🕐 **10.30am** Snack
» 1 apple and 1 tablespoon of mixed raw nuts and/or seeds

🕐 **1pm** Lunch
» Tandoori chicken salad (p124)

🕐 **4pm** Snack
» 1 small fat-free Greek yoghurt with half a pack of berries

🕐 **7pm** Dinner
» Ratatouille with 1 small baked sweet potato (p125)

4-week total body blitz workout plan

» Rest day, all levels

4-week total body blitz diet plan

Day 11

🕐 **7.30am** Breakfast
» 1 green pineapple juice (p120)
» Supplements

🕐 **10.30am** Snack
» 1 apple and 1 tablespoon of mixed raw nuts and/or seeds

🕐 **1pm** Lunch
» Tuna Niçoise salad (p124)

🕐 **4pm** Snack
» 1 small fat-free Greek yoghurt with half a pack of berries

🕐 **7pm** Dinner
» Falafel (p128) with cauliflower 'couscous' (p126) and beetroot dip (p124)

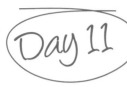

4-week workout plan

Repeat circuit from day 4 (p101) using these reps and sets:

Plus
» Interval training

Beginner	Intermediate	Advanced
1-min walk	2-min jog	1-min jog
1-min jog	1-min sprint	1-min run
x18	**x12**	1-min sprint
		x12

🕐 **8.30am** Lower-body toning session

Beginner: Choose 4 exercises, perform each for 35 secs; complete 2 circuits

Intermediate: Choose 5 exercises, perform each for 50 secs; complete 2 circuits

Advanced: Perform all exercises for 70 secs each; complete 2 circuits

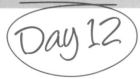

Day 12

4-week total body blitz diet plan

🕐 **7.30am** Breakfast
» 1 tomato and celery juice (p120)
» Supplements

🕐 **10.30am** Snack
» 1 apple and 1 tablespoon of mixed raw nuts and/or seeds

🕐 **1pm** Lunch
» Egg salad (p127) with tofu mayonnaise (p126)

🕐 **4pm** Snack
» 1 small fat-free Greek yoghurt with half a pack of berries

🕐 **7pm** Dinner
» Lentil soup (p130)

4-week total body blitz workout plan

🕐 **6pm** 1-hour cardio or class, all levels

4-week total body blitz diet plan

🕐 **7.30am** Breakfast
» 1 morning refresher juice (p120)
» Supplements

🕐 **10.30am** Snack
» 1 apple and 1 tablespoon of mixed raw nuts and/or seeds

🕐 **1pm** Lunch
» Salmon fillet salad (p130)

🕐 **4pm** Snack
» 1 small fat-free Greek yoghurt with half a pack of berries

🕐 **7pm** Dinner
» Roast pork with Puy lentils (p128)

4-week total body blitz workout plan

🕐 **9am** Repeat circuit from day 6 (p104)

Beginner: 35 secs each exercise, repeat 4 times

Intermediate: 50 secs each exercise, repeat 4 times

Advanced: 70 secs each exercise, repeat 4 times

Plus
» Interval training

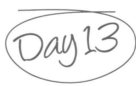

Day 13

Beginner	Intermediate	Advanced
1-min walk	2-min jog	1-min jog
1-min jog	1-min sprint	1-min run
x18	**x12**	1-min sprint
		x12

4-week total body blitz diet plan

🕐 **7.30am** Breakfast
» 1 vitamin vitality juice (p120)
» Supplements

🕐 **10.30am** Snack
» 1 apple and 1 tablespoon of mixed raw nuts and/or seeds

🕐 **1pm** Lunch
» Feta and mint salad (p124)

🕐 **4pm** Snack
» 1 small fat-free Greek yoghurt with half a pack of berries

🕐 **7pm** Dinner
» Ratatouille with 1 small baked sweet potato (p125)

4-week total body blitz workout plan

🕐 **6pm** 1-hour Pilates class or DVD, all levels

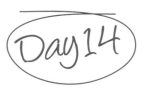

Day 14

4-week total body blitz diet plan

week **3**

🕐 **7am** Lemon cleanse
» 1 glass room-temperature water with lemon

🕐 **7.30am** Breakfast
» 1 beetroot liver cleanse juice (p120)
» Supplements

🕐 **10.30am** Snack
» 1 apple and 2 tablespoons of mixed raw nuts or seeds

🕐 **1pm** Lunch
» Green goddess soup (p122)

🕐 **4pm** Snack
» 2 tablespoons of mixed raw nuts or seeds and 2 handfuls of blueberries

🕐 **7pm** Dinner
» Cauliflower detox soup (p122)

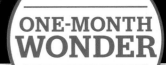

ONE-MONTH WONDER

Day 15

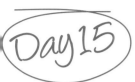
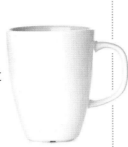

🕙 **10pm** Overnight detox drink
» 1 cup of instant miso soup

4-week total body blitz workout plan

🕔 **5pm** Skipping workout

Beginner	Intermediate	Advanced
Skip 30 secs	Skip 40 secs	Skip 45 secs
March on the spot 30 secs	March on the spot 20 secs	March on the spot 15 secs
x15	x15	x15

Plus
» Repeat day 1 upper-body circuit (p94)

Reps and sets:
Beginner: Choose 5 exercises and complete 3 circuits, performing each exercise for 35 secs

Intermediate: Choose 7 exercises and complete 3 circuits, performing each exercise for 50 secs

Advanced: Complete 3 circuits of all exercises, performing each exercise for 70 secs

4-week total body blitz diet plan

🕢 **7.30am** Breakfast
» 1 breakfast boost juice (p121)
» Supplements

🕥 **10.30am** Snack
» 1 apple and 1 tablespoon of mixed raw nuts and/or seeds

🕐 **1pm** Lunch
» Cottage cheese salad with 1 small wholemeal roll (p128)

🕓 **4pm** Snack
» 1 small fat-free Greek yoghurt with half a pack of berries

🕖 **7pm** Dinner
» Chicken stir-fry with 1 cup cooked brown rice (p126)

Day 16

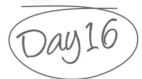

4-week total body blitz workout plan

🕗 **8am** Core and tummy toning session

» Repeat day 2 circuit (p98)

Reps and sets:
Twisting crunch
Beginner: 2 sets of 14 (7 twists each side)
Intermediate: 2 sets of 16 (8 twists each side)
Advanced: 3 sets of 20 (10 twists each side)

Reverse crunch
Beginner: 2 sets of 12
Intermediate: 3 sets of 15
Advanced: 3 sets of 20

Russian twist
Beginner: 2 sets of 12

Intermediate: 2 sets of 15
Advanced: 2 sets of 20

Knee lift
Beginner: 2 sets of 15 (1-sec hold)
Intermediate: 2 set of 15 (2-sec hold)
Advanced: 2 sets of 15 (3-sec hold)

Hip bridge
Beginner: 2 sets of 12
Intermediate: 2 sets of 15
Advanced: 2 sets of 20

4-week total body blitz diet plan

🕐 **7.30am** Breakfast
» 1 vitamin vitality juice (p120)
» Supplements

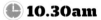 *Day 17*

🕐 **10.30am** Snack
» 1 apple and 1 tablespoon of mixed raw nuts and/or seeds

🕐 **1pm** Lunch
» Tandoori chicken salad (p124) with 1 cup of quinoa tabouleh (p130)

🕐 **4pm** Snack
» 1 small fat-free Greek yoghurt with half a pack of berries

🕐 **7pm** Dinner
» Ratatouille with 1 small baked sweet potato (p125)

workout plan

» Rest day, all levels

4-week total body blitz diet plan

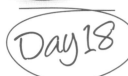 *Day 18*

🕐 **7.30am** Breakfast
» 1 green pineapple juice (p120)
» Supplements

🕐 **10.30am** Snack
» 1 apple and 1 tablespoon of raw nuts and/or seeds

🕐 **1pm** Lunch
» Tuna Niçoise salad (p124) with 1 cup of kidney beans

🕐 **4pm** Snack
» 1 fat-free Greek yoghurt with half a pack of berries

🕐 **7pm** Dinner
» Vegetable pasta (p128)

workout plan

🕐 **5pm** Lower-body toning session

» Repeat day 4 circuit (p101) using these reps and sets:

Beginner: Choose 4 exercises, perform each for 35 secs; complete 3 circuits

Intermediate: Choose 5 exercises, perform each for 50 secs; complete 3 circuits

Advanced: Perform all exercises for 70 secs each; complete 3 circuits

Plus
🕐 **6pm** Interval training

Beginner	Intermediate	Advanced
1-min walk	2-min jog	1-min jog
1-min jog	1-min sprint	1-min run
x20	**x14**	1-min sprint
		x14

4-week total body blitz diet plan

🕐 **7.30am** Breakfast
» 1 tomato and celery juice (p120)
» Supplements

🕐 **10.30am** Snack
» 1 apple and 1 tablespoon of mixed raw nuts and/or seeds

🕐 **1pm** Lunch
» Salmon fillet salad (p130)

🕐 **4pm** Snack
» 1 small fat-free Greek yoghurt with half a pack of berries

🕐 **7pm** Dinner
» Lentil soup (p130) with 1 small wholemeal roll

4-week total body blitz workout plan

🕐 **8am** 1-hour cardio or class, all levels

Day 19

4-week total body blitz diet plan

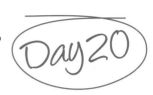
Day 20

🕐 **7.30am** Breakfast
» 1 morning refresher juice (p120)
» Supplements

🕐 **10.30am** Snack
» 1 apple and 1 tablespoon of mixed raw nuts and/or seeds

🕐 **1pm** Lunch
» Cottage cheese salad (p128)

🕐 **4pm** Snack
» 1 small fat-free Greek yoghurt with half a pack of berries

🕐 **7pm** Dinner
» Vegetable chilli with 1 cup brown rice (p130)

4-week total body blitz workout plan

🕐 **5pm** Repeat day 6 circuit (p104) using these reps and sets

Beginner: 40 secs each exercise, repeat 4 times

Intermediate: 55 secs each exercise, repeat 4 times

Advanced: 75 secs each exercise, repeat 4 times

Plus
» Interval training

Beginner	Intermediate	Advanced
1-min walk	2-min jog	1-min jog
1-min jog	1-min sprint	1-min run
x20	**x14**	1-min sprint
		x14

4-week total body blitz diet plan

🕐 **7.30am** Breakfast
» 1 breakfast boost juice (p121)
» Supplements

🕐 **10.30am** Snack
» 1 apple and 1 tablespoon of mixed raw nuts and/or seeds

🕐 **1pm** Lunch
» Feta and mint salad (p124) with 1 slice pumpernickel bread

🕐 **4pm** Snack
» 1 small fat-free Greek yoghurt with half a pack of berries

🕐 **7pm** Dinner
» Ratatouille with 1 small baked sweet potato (p125)

workout plan

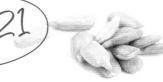

🕐 **6pm** 1-hour Pilates class or DVD, all levels

Day 21

---

week **4**

...Nearly finished!

4-week total body blitz diet plan

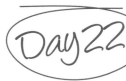

Day 22

🕐 **7am**
Lemon cleanse
» 1 glass of room-temperature water with a squeeze of lemon

🕐 **7.30am**
Breakfast
» 1 beetroot liver cleanse juice (p120)
» Supplements

🕐 **10.30am**
Snack
» 1 apple and 2 tablespoons raw nuts and/or seeds

🕐 **1pm** Lunch
» Green goddess soup (p122)

🕐 **4pm** Snack
» 2 tablespoons of mixed raw nuts or seeds and 2 handfuls of blueberries

🕐 **7pm** Dinner
» Cauliflower soup (p122)

🕐 **10pm** Overnight detox drink
» 1 cup of instant miso soup

workout plan

🕐 **5pm** Skipping workout

Beginner	Intermediate	Advanced
Skip 30 secs	Skip 40 secs	Skip 45 secs
March on the spot 30 secs	March on the spot 20 secs	March on the spot 15 secs
x17	x17	x17

Plus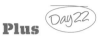

» Repeat day 1 circuit (p94)

Reps and sets:

Beginner: Choose 5 exercises and complete 3 circuits, performing each exercise for 40 secs

Intermediate: Choose 7 exercises and complete 3 circuits, performing each exercise for 60 secs

Advanced: Complete all exercises and complete 3 circuits, performing each exercise for 75 secs

workout plan *Day 23*

🕘 **9am** Repeat day 2 circuit (p98)

Reps and sets:	Reverse crunch	Intermediate:	Advanced:
Twisting crunch	**Beginner:**	3 sets of 15-20	2 sets of 15
Beginner:	2 sets of 12-15	**Advanced:**	(3-sec hold)
2 sets of 16 (8	**Intermediate:**	3 sets of 20-25	
twists each side)	3 sets of 15-20		**Hip bridge**
Intermediate:	**Advanced:**	**Knee lift**	**Beginner:**
2 sets of 18 (9	3 sets of 20-25	**Beginner:** 2 sets	2 sets of 12-15
twists each side)		of 15 (1-sec hold)	**Intermediate:**
Advanced:	**Russian twist**	**Intermediate:**	2 sets of 15-20
3 sets of 22 (11	**Beginner:**	2 set of 15	**Advanced:**
twists each side)	2 sets of 12-15	(2-sec hold)	2 sets of 20-25

4-week **total body blitz diet plan**

🕘 **7.30am**
Breakfast
» 1 slice wholemeal toast with 2 eggs
» Supplements

🕘 **10.30am**
Snack
» 1 apple and 1 tablespoon of raw nuts

🕘 **1pm** Lunch
» Feta and mint salad (p124) with quinoa tabouleh (p130)

🕘 **4pm** Snack
» 1 fat-free Greek yoghurt with berries

🕘 **7pm**
Dinner
» Falafel (p128) with cauliflower 'couscous' (p126) and beetroot dip (p124)

4-week **total body blitz diet plan**

🕘 **7.30am** Breakfast
» 1 Weetabix with skimmed milk and berries
» Supplements

🕘 **10.30am** Snack
» 1 apple and 1 tablespoon of raw nuts and/or seeds

🕘 **1pm** Lunch
» Lentil soup with 1 small wholemeal roll (p130)

🕘 **4pm** Snack
» 1 fat-free Greek yoghurt with half a pack of berries

🕘 **7pm**
Dinner
» California omelette (p126)

Day 24

workout plan

» Rest day, all levels

4-week total body blitz diet

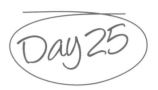

7.30am Breakfast
» 1 boiled egg with 1 slice wholemeal toast with Marmite
» Supplements

10.30am Snack
» 1 apple and 1 tablespoon of mixed raw nuts and/or seeds

1pm Lunch
» Tandoori chicken salad with half a pitta bread (p124)

4pm Snack
» 1 small fat-free Greek yoghurt with half a pack of berries

workout plan

5pm Interval training

Beginner	Intermediate	Advanced
1-min walk	2-min jog	1-min jog
1-min jog	1-min sprint	1-min run
x22	**x15**	1-min sprint
		x15

7pm Dinner
» Ratatouille with 1 small baked sweet potato (p125)

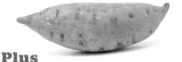

Plus
Repeat day 4 circuit (p101) with these reps and sets:

Beginner: Choose 4 exercises, perform each for 35 secs; complete 4 circuits

Intermediate: Choose 5 exercises, perform each for 50 secs; 4 circuits

Advanced: Perform all exercises for 70 secs each; complete 4 circuits

4-week total body blitz diet plan

7.30am Breakfast
» 1 cup of porridge, made with skimmed milk and served with half a pack of berries
» Supplements

10.30am Snack
» 1 apple and 1 tablespoon of mixed raw nuts and/or seeds

1pm Lunch
» Feta and mint salad with 1 cup cooked broad beans (p124)

4pm Snack
» 1 small fat-free Greek yoghurt with half a pack of berries

7pm Dinner
» Vegetable pasta (p128)

workout plan

6pm 1-hour class, all levels

4-week total body blitz diet plan

Day 27

(◷) **7.30am** Breakfast
≫ Mushroom omelette (p127)
≫ Supplements

(◷) **10.30am** Snack
≫ 1 apple and 1 tablespoon of mixed raw nuts and/or seeds

(◷) **1pm** Lunch
≫ Smoked salmon salad sandwich (p126)

(◷) **4pm** Snack
≫ 1 small fat-free Greek yoghurt with half a pack of berries

(◷) **7pm** Dinner
≫ Roast pollock with salsa verde and butter bean mash (p127)

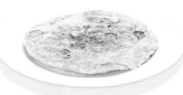

workout plan

Plus Repeat day 6 circuit (p104)

(◷) **6pm** Interval training

Beginner	Intermediate	Advanced
1-min walk	2-min jog	1-min jog
1-min jog	1-min sprint	1-min run
x22	x15	1-min sprint
		x15

Beginner: 45 secs each exercise, repeat 4 times
Intermediate: 60 secs each exercise, repeat 4 times
Advanced: 80 secs each exercise, repeat 4 times

4-week total body blitz diet plan

(◷) **7.30am** Breakfast
≫ 1 Weetabix with skimmed milk and half a pack berries
≫ Supplements

(◷) **10.30am** Snack
≫ 1 apple and 1 tablespoon of mixed raw nuts and/or seeds

(◷) **1pm** Lunch
≫ Cottage cheese salad (p128) with 1 small wholemeal roll

(◷) **4pm** Snack
≫ 1 small fat-free Greek yoghurt with half a pack of berries

(◷) **7pm** Dinner
≫ Chicken stir-fry with 1 cup of cooked brown rice (p126)

workout plan

Day 28

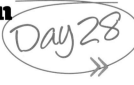

(◷) **9am** 1-hour Pilates class, all levels

Your results

Track your progress on the 4-week total body blitz

	Before	After 1 week	After 2 weeks	After 3 weeks	After 4 weeks
Weight					
Arms					
Bust					
Waist					
Hips					
Thighs					

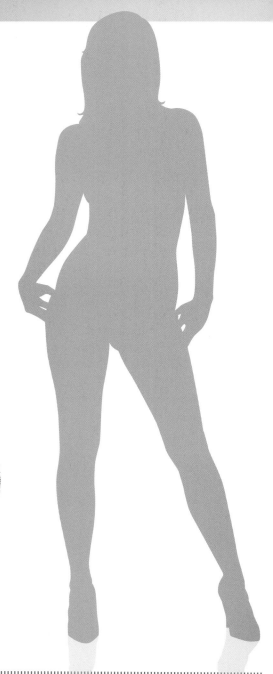

Congratulations, you did it! We hope you feel fantastic!

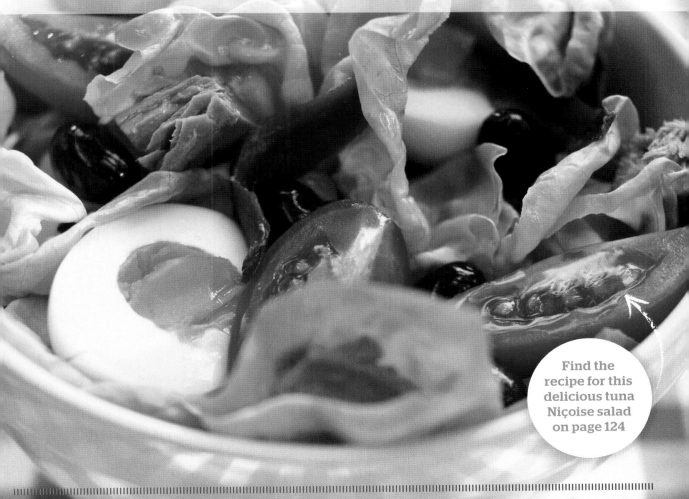

Recipes

Find the recipe for this delicious tuna Niçoise salad on page 124

Juices

Kick-start your mornings with these healthy, cleansing combinations

Method
» Put the ingredients through a juicer and drink immediately
» All recipes make 2 servings

Green pineapple juice

1 bunch watercress
1 bunch parsley
4 broccoli florets
1 celery stick
½ pineapple, peeled

Tomato and celery juice

6 tomatoes
2 celery sticks
½ red pepper

Vitamin vitality juice

8 tomatoes
7 carrots, trimmed
2 celery sticks
½ cucumber
1 handful
cabbage leaves
½ yellow pepper
1 garlic clove, peeled
½ onion, peeled

Morning refresher juice

2 apples
1 lemon, peeled
1 handful fresh mint

Sunrise juice

2 oranges, peeled
½ cantaloupe melon
1 nectarine

Beetroot liver cleanse juice

4 carrots
3 celery sticks
½ cucumber
1 small beetroot, chopped

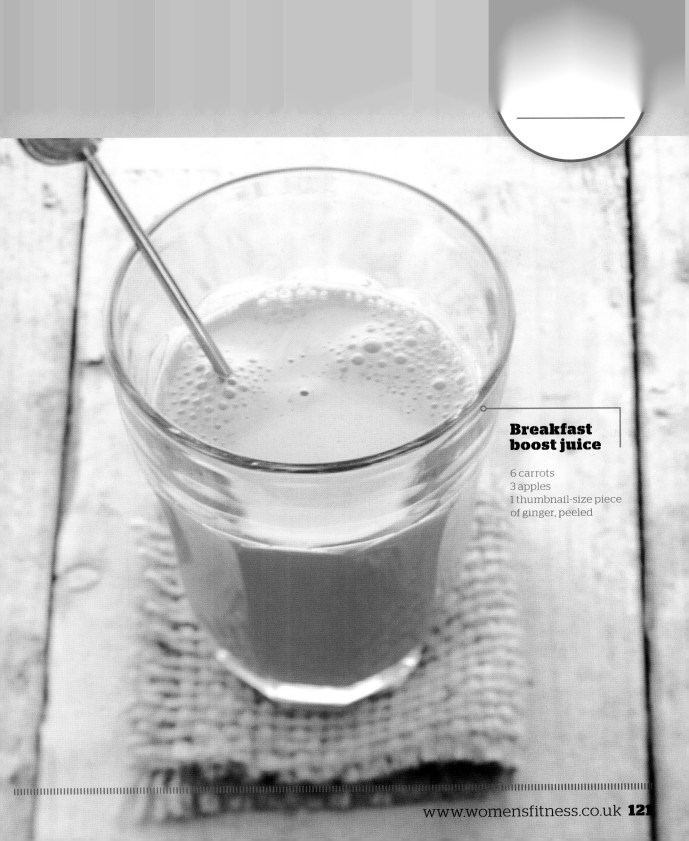

Breakfast boost juice

6 carrots
3 apples
1 thumbnail-size piece
of ginger, peeled

Soups

Cook up these healthy, easy soups to get great results

Note
» All recipes serve 4

Green goddess soup

Extra virgin olive oil cooking spray
1 onion, chopped
1 garlic clove, crushed
750ml vegetable stock
2 turnips, trimmed, scrubbed
and chopped
2 courgettes, chopped
200g kale, roughly chopped
Salt and pepper
1 handful fresh, chopped dill

» Mist a non-stick saucepan with the
olive oil cooking spray. Fry the onion
for 5 minutes then add the garlic and
fry for 1 minute. Add the stock and
turnips and simmer for 10 minutes.
Then add the courgettes and kale
and cook for 5 minutes. Purée using
a hand blender, season to taste then
serve garnished with dill.

Lovely lettuce soup

Extra virgin olive oil cooking spray
1 onion, chopped
1 garlic clove, crushed
750ml vegetable stock
450g potatoes, peeled and cubed
1 romaine lettuce, leaves torn
Salt and pepper
4tbsp fresh, chopped parsley

» Mist a non-stick saucepan with
the cooking spray. Fry the onion
for 5 minutes, add the garlic and fry
for 1 minute. Pour in the stock and
add the potatoes. Bring to the boil
and simmer for 15 minutes. Add
the lettuce leaves and cook for 2
minutes until wilted. Purée using a
hand blender, season to taste then
serve garnished with parsley.

Cauliflower detox soup

Extra virgin olive oil cooking spray
2 garlic cloves, crushed
2 onions, chopped
2 cauliflower heads, chopped
1l vegetable stock
1tsp ground cumin
Squeeze of lemon juice
Salt and pepper
3tbsp fresh, chopped parsley

» Mist a non-stick saucepan with the
cooking spray. Gently fry the onion
for 5 minutes, then add the garlic
and fry for 1 minute. Add the rest of
the ingredients except the lemon
and parsley. Bring to the boil and
simmer for 15 minutes until the
cauliflower is tender. Purée the soup
using a hand blender until smooth.
Add the lemon juice and season to
taste. Serve garnished with parsley.

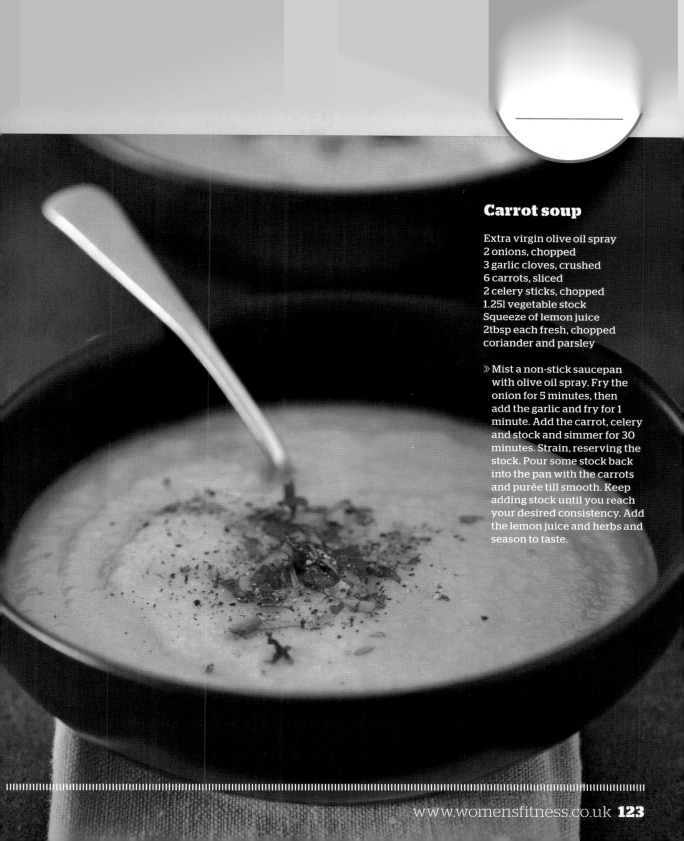

Carrot soup

Extra virgin olive oil spray
2 onions, chopped
3 garlic cloves, crushed
6 carrots, sliced
2 celery sticks, chopped
1.25l vegetable stock
Squeeze of lemon juice
2tbsp each fresh, chopped
coriander and parsley

» Mist a non-stick saucepan
with olive oil spray. Fry the
onion for 5 minutes, then
add the garlic and fry for 1
minute. Add the carrot, celery
and stock and simmer for 30
minutes. Strain, reserving the
stock. Pour some stock back
into the pan with the carrots
and purée till smooth. Keep
adding stock until you reach
your desired consistency. Add
the lemon juice and herbs and
season to taste.

Meals

Restore your energy levels and give your body a boost with a tasty, filling dish

Note

Tuna Niçoise salad

1 handful salad leaves
1 handful cherry tomatoes, halved
1 boiled egg, quartered
½ large can tuna in brine
4 anchovies, drained and blotted on kitchen paper
1tbsp extra virgin olive oil
2tsp lemon juice
Salt and pepper

>> Arrange all the salad ingredients on a plate. Combine the olive oil and lemon juice and drizzle over the salad. Season to taste.

Beetroot dip

2tbsp tofu mayonnaise (page 126) or fat-free Greek yoghurt
½ small, cooked beetroot
Freshly ground black pepper
Squeeze of lemon juice

» Combine all the ingredients in a blender and process until smooth.

Feta and mint salad

1 large handful salad leaves
2tbsp frozen peas, steamed and cooled
100g feta
2tbsp chopped fresh mint
1tbsp extra virgin olive oil
2tsp lemon juice

» Arrange the salad leaves on a plate, scatter with the peas and crumble over the feta. Sprinkle with the fresh mint. Combine the olive oil and lemon juice and drizzle over the salad to serve.

Tandoori chicken salad

1tbsp fat-free Greek yoghurt
1tsp tikka masala paste
Squeeze of lemon juice
1 skinless chicken breast
1 large handful salad leaves

» Preheat the oven to 200°C/400°F/ Gas Mark 6. Combine the yoghurt, tikka masala paste and lemon juice. Coat the chicken with the yoghurt mix and refrigerate for at least 20 minutes. Put a baking tray in the oven for 5 minutes. Place the chicken on the tray and bake for 20-25 minutes or until cooked through. Serve with salad leaves and 2 tablespoons of homemade tzatziki (page 130).

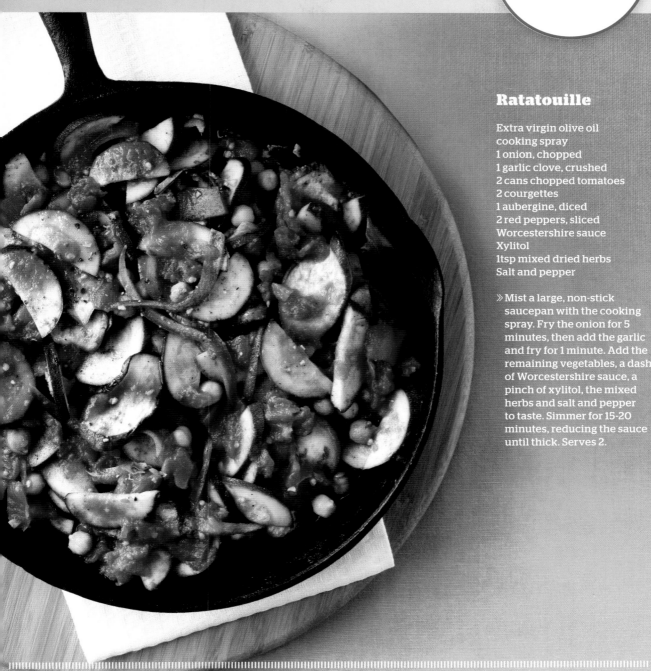

Ratatouille

Extra virgin olive oil
cooking spray
1 onion, chopped
1 garlic clove, crushed
2 cans chopped tomatoes
2 courgettes
1 aubergine, diced
2 red peppers, sliced
Worcestershire sauce
Xylitol
1tsp mixed dried herbs
Salt and pepper

» Mist a large, non-stick
saucepan with the cooking
spray. Fry the onion for 5
minutes, then add the garlic
and fry for 1 minute. Add the
remaining vegetables, a dash
of Worcestershire sauce, a
pinch of xylitol, the mixed
herbs and salt and pepper
to taste. Simmer for 15-20
minutes, reducing the sauce
until thick. Serves 2.

Chicken stir-fry

Extra virgin olive oil cooking spray
1 chicken breast, diced
Soya sauce
½ head broccoli, cut into small florets
1 handful sugar snap peas
4 baby corn spears
1tbsp oyster sauce

» Mist a wok with cooking spray. Stir-fry the chicken for 2 minutes, then add a dash of soya sauce and a little water, place a lid over the pan and cook until chicken is done. Remove the chicken and keep warm. Cook the broccoli, covered, for 5 minutes, then add the remaining veggies. Drain any water, return the chicken to the pan, stir through the oyster sauce and serve.

Smoked salmon sandwich

2 thin slices rye or spelt bread
2tsp low-fat soft cheese
1 handful rocket
100g smoked salmon
Squeeze of lemon juice
Freshly ground black pepper
1tbsp dill, chopped

» Spread the bread with the cheese and layer the rocket and salmon on one slice. Squeeze over lemon juice, season with pepper and add the dill. Top with the other slice and serve.

California omelette

Extra virgin olive oil cooking spray
2 eggs
1 tomato, chopped
½ avocado, sliced
1 handful alfalfa sprouts
1 sprig coriander, chopped
Squeeze of lime juice

» Mist a non-stick frying pan with the cooking spray and heat to smoking point. Beat the eggs, then pour into the pan and cook for 2-3 minutes. Top with the remaining ingredients and flip over. Serve immediately.

Tofu mayonnaise

180g silken tofu
1tbsp extra virgin olive oil
2 garlic cloves
1 large handful basil leaves
Salt and pepper

>> Put all the ingredients in a blender and process until smooth. You could also add anchovies, horseradish or other herbs for a different flavour, if desired.

Cauliflower pizza

1 cauliflower, broken into florets
2 egg whites, lightly beaten
1tbsp grated Parmesan cheese
1tsp mixed dried herbs
1 garlic clove, crushed
Extra virgin olive oil cooking spray
2tbsp reduced-fat tomato pasta sauce
Mixed sliced vegetables (eg: courgette, pepper, onion, carrot)
1tbsp capers, rinsed

» Preheat the oven to 200°C/400°F/ Gas Mark 6. Steam the cauliflower until tender, then place in a bowl and use a hand blender to process until almost smooth. Add the egg whites, cheese, herbs and garlic. Pour into a shallow tin or baking tray misted with cooking spray. Bake for 20 minutes until browned at the edges. Remove, top with pasta sauce, mixed vegetables and capers and bake for 10-15 minutes. Serve.

Cauliflower 'couscous'

1 cauliflower, roughly chopped
1 handful each fresh coriander, mint and parsley, roughly chopped
Juice of ½ lemon
1 chilli, deseeded
Salt and pepper

» Combine all the ingredients in a blender and process to a crumb consistency. Serve.

Pollock with salsa verde and butter bean mash

Extra virgin olive oil cooking spray
2 x 100g fillets pollock or other firm, white fish
Salt and pepper

Salsa verde
2tbsp extra virgin olive oil
1 large handful baby spinach leaves
1 small bunch flat-leaf parsley, leaves picked
1 sprig each mint and oregano
1tbsp capers, drained
1tsp dijon mustard
Squeeze of lemon juice

Butter bean mash
Extra virgin olive oil cooking spray
1 onion, finely chopped
1 garlic clove, crushed
¼tsp turmeric
1 tin butter beans, drained and rinsed
Squeeze of lemon juice

» Preheat the oven to 180°C/350°F/Gas Mark 4. Mist a large piece of foil with cooking spray and place the fish on top. Season. Seal the edges of the foil to make an airtight parcel and bake for 15-20 minutes until cooked through. Meanwhile, put all the salsa verde ingredients in a blender and process until almost smooth. Cover and put in the fridge. To make the mash, mist a non-stick saucepan with cooking spray and gently fry the onion and garlic till softened. Add the turmeric, butter beans and 2 tablespoons of water. Simmer until heated through. Use a hand blender to process till smooth. Stir through the lemon juice. Divide the mash between 2 plates and top each with a fish fillet and the salsa verde. Serves 2.

Egg salad

1 handful salad leaves
6 cherry tomatoes
2 poached eggs
1tsp chopped chives
1tbsp extra virgin olive oil
2tsp lemon juice
Salt and pepper

>> Arrange the mixed leaves and tomatoes on a plate. Top with poached eggs and sprinkle with chives. Combine the olive oil and lemon juice and drizzle over the salad. Season to taste and serve.

Prawn skewers

2 garlic cloves, crushed
1tbsp olive oil
1tbsp lemon juice
200g raw, peeled prawns
1tbsp chopped parsley
Mixed salad leaves, to serve

» Combine the garlic, olive oil and lemon juice and toss through the prawns. Cover and refrigerate for 20 minutes. Preheat a grill and thread the prawns onto skewers. Grill for 3-5 minutes on each side until cooked through. Sprinkle with parsley and serve on a bed of mixed salad leaves. Serves 2.

Mushroom omelette

Extra virgin olive oil cooking spray
1 garlic clove, crushed
8 button mushrooms, thinly sliced
1 egg and 2 egg whites, beaten
1tbsp grated Parmesan cheese
1tbsp chopped parsley

» Mist a non-stick frying pan with cooking spray, then gently fry the garlic and mushrooms. When softened, add the egg mixture and increase the heat to medium high. Cook for 2-3 minutes until the eggs are set. Remove from the heat, sprinkle over the cheese and parsley, flip the omelette in half and serve immediately.

Stuffed mushrooms

Extra virgin olive oil cooking spray
2-3 Portobello mushrooms
1 large tomato, chopped
50g feta cheese, crumbled
1 handful parsley, chopped

» Preheat the oven to 200°C/400°F/
Gas Mark 6. Mist a baking tray with
cooking spray. Remove the stalks of
the mushrooms and chop. Combine
with the tomato, feta and parsley
and pile the mixture on top of the
mushrooms. Place on the baking
tray and bake for 10-15 minutes
until golden.

Vegetable pasta

½ jar reduced-fat pasta sauce
½ courgette, sliced
½ red and ½ yellow pepper, sliced
Tabasco sauce
Soya sauce
75g wholewheat pasta
1 handful parsley, chopped

» Heat the pasta sauce in a saucepan
over medium heat. Add the
courgette and pepper and simmer
for 10-15 minutes until tender.
Add a dash of Tabasco and soya
sauce. Meanwhile, cook the pasta
according to packet directions.
Pour the sauce over the pasta and
garnish with the parsley to serve.

Falafel

Extra virgin olive oil cooking spray
½ red onion, finely chopped
1 garlic clove, crushed
½ can chickpeas, drained and rinsed
Pinch each cumin, ground coriander
and cayenne pepper
½tbsp chickpea flour
1tbsp coriander, chopped
1 egg, lightly beaten

» Preheat the oven to 180°C/350°F/
Gas Mark 4. Mist a baking tray with
cooking spray. Mix the remaining
ingredients to form a dough, adding
a little water if needed. Roll into
balls. Place on the prepared baking
tray and bake for 15-20 minutes.

Cottage cheese salad

1 large handful salad leaves
2 radishes, finely sliced
100g low-fat cottage cheese
1tbsp chives, chopped

>> Arrange the salad leaves
and radishes on a plate.
Top with the cottage
cheese and sprinkle
with chives to serve.

Roast pork with Puy lentils

Extra virgin olive oil cooking spray
1tsp each ground coriander
and turmeric
2 garlic cloves, crushed
1tsp freshly grated ginger
Freshly ground black pepper
1tsp extra virgin olive oil
2 lean pork steaks, fat removed

Puy lentils
½ onion, chopped
100g Puy lentils
600ml vegetable stock
½ stick celery, finely chopped
½tsp each turmeric, ground
coriander and cumin
½tsp freshly grated ginger
1 garlic clove, crushed
½ red chilli, deseeded, finely chopped

» Preheat the oven to 180°C/350°F/
Gas Mark 4. Mist a baking tray with
cooking spray. Mix the spices, garlic,
ginger and pepper with the olive
oil and brush over the pork steaks.
Place on the baking tray and bake
for 15-20 minutes.
» Meanwhile, for the Puy lentils, mist
a large, non-stick saucepan with the
cooking spray. Add the onion and
fry for 5 minutes. Add the lentils
and stock and simmer for 15-20
minutes until lentils are tender. Add
remaining ingredients and simmer
for 5 minutes. Serve the pork on a
bed of lentils and accompany with
steamed vegetables. Serves 2.

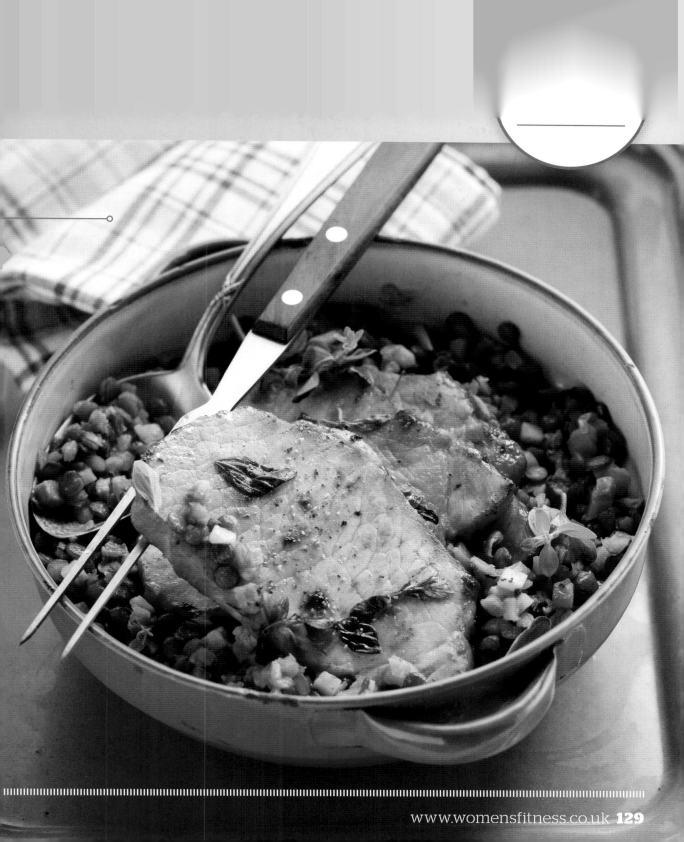

Salmon fillet salad

1 salmon fillet
½ bag baby spinach leaves
1tbsp pine nuts, toasted
1tbsp extra virgin olive oil
2tsp lemon juice

» Steam the salmon until cooked through. Arrange the spinach leaves on a plate, top with the salmon and sprinkle over the pine nuts. Combine the olive oil and lemon juice and drizzle over the salad to serve.

Quinoa tabouleh

100g quinoa, cooked and cooled
1tbsp pistachio kernels, chopped
1 lemon, juiced
Pinch each cayenne pepper, cumin and ground coriander
Seeds of ½ pomegranate
Salt and pepper

>> Combine all the ingredients and mix well.

Vegetable chilli

Extra virgin olive oil cooking spray
1 onion, chopped
1 garlic clove, crushed
1 red chilli, deseeded, finely chopped
1 celery stick, finely sliced
1 green pepper, chopped
1 tin red kidney beans, drained
250ml passata

» Mist a non-stick saucepan with cooking spray. Fry the onion for 5 minutes. Add the garlic and fry for 1 minute. Add the remaining ingredients and simmer for 15-20 minutes until the vegetables are tender. Serves 2.

Cod with stir-fried vegetables

Extra virgin olive oil cooking spray
1 fillet cod or other firm, white fish
1tbsp soya sauce
1tsp mirin or sherry
1 garlic clove, crushed
1tsp freshly grated ginger
Mixed stir-fried vegetables, to serve

» Preheat the oven to 180°C/350°F/ Gas Mark 4. Mist a piece of foil with cooking spray and place the cod on top. Combine the soya, mirin, garlic and ginger and pour over the fish. Fold up the foil to form an airtight parcel. Bake for 20 minutes. Serve with stir-fried vegetables.

Lentil soup

Extra virgin olive oil cooking spray
1 onion, chopped
1 garlic clove, crushed
Pinch each cumin and ground coriander
1 carrot, sliced
75g red lentils
500ml vegetable stock
Salt and pepper
Squeeze of lemon juice

» Mist a non-stick saucepan with cooking spray. Fry the onion for 5 minutes, then add the garlic and fry for 1 minute. Add the rest of the ingredients except the lemon juice. Simmer for 30-35 minutes. Use a hand blender to process till smooth. Season to taste and add the lemon juice. Serves 2.

Tzatziki

1 small tub fat-free Greek yoghurt
¼ cucumber, grated
Squeeze of lemon
1 handful mint leaves, chopped

» Combine all the ingredients and chill.